D1627860

Soccer Fitness:

A Step-by-Step Guide on Speed, Endurance, Flexibility, and Strength for a Soccer Player

Dylan Joseph

Soccer Fitness:
A Step-by-Step Guide on Speed, Endurance, Flexibility, and
Strength for a Soccer Player

By: Dylan Joseph

© 2021
All Rights Reserved

WAIT!

Wouldn't it be nice to have an easy one-page FREE PDF printout with off-season and in-season workouts discussed in this book? Well, here is your chance!

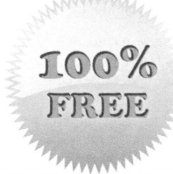

UNDERSTANDSOCCER.COM - WEIGHT TRAINING WORKOUTS

Weight Training - Off-Season

Monday - Upper Body Pull

Exercise	Sets	Reps	Workout 1	Workout 2	Workout 3
Pull-Ups	3	Max			
Rows	3	5-6			
Hip Huggers	3	5-6			
*Dumbbell Curls	3	6-8			
Leg Raises	3	Max			

Wednesday - Lower Body

Exercise	Sets	Reps	Workout 1	Workout 2	Workout 3
Bench Presses	3	5-6			
Dips	3	Max			
Overhead Presses	3	5-6			
*Triceps Extensions	3	6-8			
Sit-Ups	3	Max			

Friday - Upper Body Push

Exercise	Sets	Reps	Workout 1	Workout 2	Workout 3
Squats	3	5-6			
Deadlifts	3	5-6			
Lunges	3	6-8			
Calf Raises	3	12-15			
Planks	3	Max			

*Optional exercise for a smaller body part. Take sets to failure
Perform a warm-up that includes warm-up sets of exercises above with reduced weight.

Weight Training - During Season

1-2X per Week

Exercise	Sets	Reps	Workout 1	Workout 2	Workout 3
Squat	2	5-6			
Deadlift	2	5-6			
Calf Raises	2	12-15			
Bench Press	2	5-6			
Pull-Ups	2	Max			
Overhead Press	2	5-6			
Rows	2	5-6			
Sit-Ups	2	Max			
Leg Raises	2	Max			

Go to this Link for an **Instant** One-Page Printout:
UnderstandSoccer.com/free-printout

This FREE workout log is simply a thank you for purchasing this book. This PDF printout will ensure that you have a terrific workout to perform to get you ready for the soccer field!

Soccer Fitness:
A Step-by-Step Guide on Speed, Endurance, Flexibility, and Strength
for a Soccer Player
All Rights Reserved
July 9, 2021
Copyright © 2021 Understand, LLC
Dylan@UnderstandSoccer.com
Printed in the United States of America

No part of this book may be reproduced or transmitted in any form or by any means, electronic or mechanical, including, but not limited to photocopying, recording or by any information storage and retrieval system, without the permission in writing from Understand, LLC. The information provided within this book is for general informational and educational purposes only and does not constitute an endorsement of any websites or other sources. If you apply ideas contained in this book, you are taking full responsibility for your actions. There are no representations or warranties, express or implied, about the completeness, accuracy, reliability, suitability, or availability concerning the information, products, or services contained in this book for any purpose. The author does not assume and hereby disclaims all liability to any party for any loss, damage, or disruption caused by errors or omissions, whether the errors or omissions result from accident, negligence, or any other cause.

Any use of this information is at your own risk. The methods described in this book are the author's personal thoughts. They are not intended to be a definitive set of instructions for everyone. You may discover there are other methods and materials suitable to accomplish the same result. This book contains information that is intended to help the readers be better-informed consumers of soccer knowledge. Always consult your physician for your individual needs before beginning any new exercise program. This book is not intended to be a substitute for the medical advice of a licensed physician.

Table of Contents

Dedication

This book is dedicated to you, the soccer player, who cares so much about succeeding that you are willing to read a book to improve your fitness to help improve your soccer game. Learning is exceptionally noble and speaks volumes to the person you are.

Also, this book is dedicated to Tony Horton who has helped me develop a passion for fitness and training. His workout programs have helped me become muscular and fit, while helping me gain the confidence I so badly needed in high school. His guidance has been huge in helping me become a better person. For him, I am very thankful.

Preface

Being strong, having speed, and being able to avoid injury can be the difference from an average season and being the MVP on your soccer team. This book gives you the tips, tricks, tweaks, and techniques to become twice as fit as you currently are right now. Knowing when, how, and what to train when working out can make all the difference for you to succeed on the soccer field.

INDIVIDUAL SOCCER PLAYER'S PYRAMID

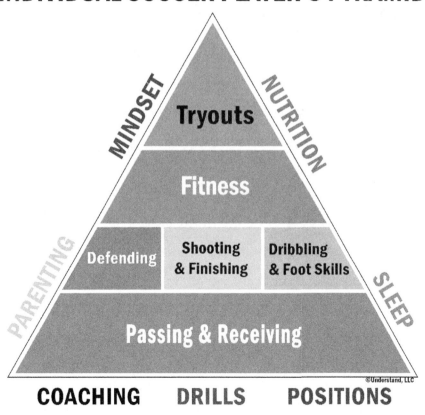

If you are looking to improve your skills, your child's confidence, or your players' abilities, then it is essential to understand where this book fits into the bigger picture of developing a soccer player. In the image, the most critical field-specific skills to work on are at the base of the Individual Soccer Player's Pyramid. This pyramid is a quality outline to improve an individual soccer player's game. All the elements in the pyramid, and the items surrounding it, play a meaningful part in becoming a better player, but certain skills should be read and mastered first before moving on to the others.

You will notice that passing and receiving is at the foundation of the pyramid. This is because if you can receive and make a pass in soccer, then you will be a useful teammate. Even though you may not consistently score, dispossess the other team, or dribble through several opponents, you will still have the fundamental tools needed to play the sport and contribute to your team.

As you move one layer up, you find yourself with a decision to make on how to progress. Specifically, the pyramid is created with you in mind because each soccer player and each soccer position have different needs. Therefore, your choice regarding which path to take first is dictated by the position you play and more importantly, by the position that you want to play. In soccer and life, just because you are in a particular spot, position, or even a job, it does not mean that you must stay there forever if that is not your choice. However, it is not recommended to refuse playing a position if you are not in the exact role you want. It takes time to develop the skills that will allow you to make a shift from one position to another.

If you want to become a forward, then consider starting your route on the second layer of the pyramid with shooting and finishing. As your abilities to shoot increase, your coach will notice your new finishing skills and will be more likely to move you up the field (if you are not a forward already). Be sure to communicate to the coach that you desire to be moved up the field to a more offensive position, which will increase your chances, as well. If you are already a forward, then dive deep into this topic to ensure you become the leading scorer; first on your team, and then in the entire league. Notice that shooting and finishing is considered to be less critical than passing and receiving. This is because you must pass the ball up the field before you can take a shot on net.

Otherwise, you can start by progressing to dribbling and foot skills from passing and receiving because the proper technique is crucial to dribble the ball well. It is often necessary for a soccer player to use a skill to protect the ball from the other team or to advance the ball up the field to place their team in a favorable situation to score. The selection of this route is often taken first by midfielders and occasionally by forwards.

Defending is another option to proceed from passing and receiving. Keeping the other team off the scoreboard is not an easy task. Developing a defender's mindset, learning which way to push a forward, understanding how to position your body, knowing when to foul, and using the correct form for headers is critical to a defender on the back line who wants to prevent goals.

Finish all three areas in the second layer of the pyramid before progressing up the pyramid. Dribbling and defending the ball (not just shooting) are useful for an attacker; shooting and defending (not just dribbling) are helpful for a midfielder, while shooting and dribbling (not just defending) are helpful for a defender. Having a well-rounded knowledge of the skills needed for the different positions is important for all soccer players. It is especially essential for those soccer players who are looking to change positions in the future. Shooting and finishing, dribbling and foot skills, as well as defending are more beneficial for soccer players to learn first, so focus on these before spending time on the upper areas of the pyramid. Also, reading about each of these areas will help you learn what your opponent wants to do.

Once you have improved your skills in the first and second tiers of the pyramid, you can move up to fitness. It is difficult to go through a passing/dribbling/finishing drill for a few minutes without being out of breath. However, as you practice everything below the fitness category in the pyramid, your fitness and strength will naturally increase. Performing technical drills allows soccer players to increase their fitness naturally. This reduces the need to focus exclusively on running for fitness.

Coming from the perspective of both a soccer player and trainer, I know that constantly focusing on running is not as fulfilling and does not create long-lasting improvements, whereas emphasizing shooting capabilities, foot skills, and defending knowledge creates long-lasting change. Often, coaches who focus on running their players in practice are also coaches who want to improve their team but have limited knowledge of many of the soccer-specific topics that would quickly increase their players' abilities. Not only does fitness in soccer include your endurance; it also addresses your ability to run with agility and speed and to develop strength and power, while using stretching to improve your flexibility. All these tools put together leads to a well-rounded soccer player.

Similar to the tier below it, you should focus on the fitness areas that will help you specifically, while keeping all the topics in mind. For example, you may be a smaller soccer player who wants to put on some muscle mass. In this case, you should emphasize weight training so that you can gain the muscle needed to avoid being pushed off the ball. However, you should still stretch before and after a lifting workout or soccer practice/game to ensure that you are limber and flexible enough to recover quickly and avoid injuries.

Maybe you are a soccer player in your 20s, 30s, or 40s. Then, emphasizing your flexibility would do a world of good to ensure you keep playing soccer for many more years. However, doing a few sets of push-ups, pull-ups, squats, lunges, sit-ups, etc. per week will help you maintain or gain a desirable physique.

Furthermore, you could be in the prime of your career in high school, college, or at the pro level, which means that obtaining the speed and endurance needed to run for 90+ minutes is the most essential key to continue pursuing your soccer aspirations.

Finally, we travel to the top of the pyramid, which involves tryouts. Although tryouts occur only 1-2 times per year, they have a huge impact on whether you will make the team or get left out of the lineup. Tryouts can cause intense anxiety if you do not know the keys to make sure that you stand out from your competitors and are very confident from the start.

If you have not read the *Understand Soccer* series book, *Soccer Training*, then it is highly recommended that you do so to gain the general knowledge of crucial topics within all the areas of the pyramid. Investing in a copy of the book will act as a good gauge to see how much you know about each topic, which will then help determine if another book in the series written about a specific subject in the soccer pyramid will be beneficial for you.

The last portion of the pyramid are the areas that surround it. Although these are not skills and topics that can be addressed by your physical abilities, they each play key roles in rounding out a complete soccer player. For example, having one or more supportive parent(s)/guardian(s) is beneficial, as they can transport the child to games, and provide the needed equipment and the fees for the team and individual training, as well as encouragement. It is also very helpful to have a quality coach whose teachings and drills will help the individual learn how their performance and skills fit into the team's big picture.

Sleeping enough is critical to having enough energy during practices and on game days, in addition to recovering from training and games. Appropriate soccer nutrition will increase a soccer player's energy and endurance, help them achieve the ideal physique, and significantly aid in their recovery.

Understanding soccer positions will help you determine if a specific role is well-suited for your skills. It is important to know there are additional types of specific positions, not just forwards, midfielders, and defenders. A former or current professional player in the same position as you can provide guidance on the requirements to effectively play that position.

Finally, you must develop a mindset that will leave you unshakable. This mindset will help you prepare for game situations, learn how to deal with others, and be mentally tough enough to not worry about situations that you cannot control, such as the condition of field, the officiating, or the weather.

The pyramid is a great visual aid to consider when choosing what areas to focus on next as a soccer player, coach, or parent. However, remember that a team's pyramid may look slightly different based on which tactics the players can handle and which approach the coach decides to use. Now that you know where this book plays into the bigger picture, let us begin.

Remember that if there are any words or terms whose meaning you are unsure of; you can feel free to reference the glossary at the back of the book.

Finally, if you enjoy this book, please leave a review on Amazon to let me know.

Introduction

Fitness often means something different for everyone. For some, it could be gaining muscle and strength; for others, it could mean becoming skinny; for others still, it could mean reducing pain, while still doing the activities that bring them joy.

Soccer Fitness was written to help you perform well in a soccer practice or game. Therefore, this book reveals how to increase your **speed**, improve your **cardiovascular endurance**, expand your muscular **strength**, grow your **muscular endurance**, enhance your **agility**, develop your **flexibility**, while reducing your **body fat** percentage to help you perform your best on the field.

With all things in the weight room and on the field, **quality (not quantity) is key**. Make sure that you do not cheat your reps to avoid injury, because the purpose of any fitness program is to improve your abilities on the field, not to injure you, which will force you to stay off the field. Exercising uses energy, so avoid working out more than once per day. Unless you have a soccer tournament, you should limit yourself to no more than one physical activity (e.g., weight training, practice, running, playing in a game, jump training, etc.) each day, while taking at least 1-2 days per week off. To obtain the most from the fitness tips in this book, **remember that good athletes**

work out, but great athletes out-work. Put in the time, effort, and education needed to grow your physical abilities past your teammates and opponents.

This book is broken into three parts:

1. Speed and Endurance
2. Weight Training
3. Stretching and Flexibility

Section on
Speed and Endurance

Chapter 1

How to Run Faster

Have you ever felt like if you became faster, that you would be a lot better at soccer? Well, this chapter is all about improving your sprinting speed. Losing foot races and not being able to sprint past defenders is frustrating. Therefore, consider these tips to sprint faster in only a short time:

1. Get your arms involved
2. Loosen your shoulders and head
3. Run on the balls of your feet
4. Practice, practice, practice

To run fast, remember that although it may seem like your lower body should do all the work, your upper body must be involved, too. Using your arms will allow you to remain balanced and propel yourself forward at a quicker rate. **Remember the saying, "Eye socket, hip pocket."** Think of your eyes in their sockets on your face, and, if you were wearing pants, where your pocket would be (near your hip). Your hands should move between these two spots on your body. While sprinting, as your hand lowers, it should travel past your "hip pocket," and, as your hand rises, it should travel up to your "eye socket."

Swing your arms in the opposite direction of your legs, so your left arm and right leg move in tandem, and your right arm and left leg do, too. Keep your elbows bent at a 65-90-degree angle throughout your sprint. Certified track coach Raymond Tucker recommends that you swing your arms at the shoulder joint, backward and forward at a 135-degree angle. Ensure that your hands are relaxed, and your fingers are open. **Many soccer players clench their fists while sprinting, but this disrupts the speed of your arms, and you will use energy to clench your fists that could be better spent by your leg muscles to run faster. Avoid swinging your arms in front of your body because it will slow you down.** Instead, pump them forward and backward.

2. Avoid shrugging with your traps to raise your shoulders. This unnecessary use of energy is better spent in your legs. Also, keep your head still while sprinting. Having your head bobbing or twisting will cause neck strain and is not proper form. Finally, keep your jaw relaxed, too. **Remember, if you are wasting effort by clenching your fist, shrugging your shoulders, or locking your jaw, you take that energy away from being better used in your arms and legs to propel you faster while sprinting.**

3. Run on the balls and toes of your feet. Landing on the balls of your foot allows you to roll quickly forward onto your toes to push off. Also, focus on having light and springy steps to reduce injury and increase speed. Keep your knees slightly bent as your foot lands, so they will bend naturally when your foot contacts the ground. Sadly, running on the balls of my feet was not something I realized I should do until I was in college but as soon as I changed my form, my speed went up dramatically.

Even the Olympic gold medalist and fastest man ever, Usain Bolt, lands and pushes off the balls of his feet. When sprinting, his foot contacts the ground briefly and quickly resumes propelling him forward. Your heel striking the ground rolls your feet from the heel to the balls of your feet, then to your toes. This is ideal for walking, but it keeps your foot on the ground too long for sprinting.

4. Practice sprinting to become better at sprinting. I made the mistake of thinking squatting and deadlifting alone would make me faster. It helped a little, but if you want to be faster, practice being faster. That means you must practice sprinting. Go to the field or track and work on 5-yard, 10-yard, and 20-yard sprints using the tips on form in this chapter to see the biggest impact on your speed.

The last thing to understand is that you can be a fast soccer player without being a fast sprinter. For the longest time, I assumed that you must be a fast sprinter to be fast in soccer, but by taking a moving first touch 95% of the time when you receive a pass, you can become a fast soccer player even if you are a slow sprinter. A moving first touch pushes the ball into space with your first touch. In a game, you should mostly be taking moving first touches because it allows you, with your first touch, to have the ball already going in the direction that you want to take it.

Often, the moving first touch is into space on the field to give yourself more time to think, pass, dribble, shoot, or whatever you need to do with the ball. **Next, by taking the first step with your moving first touch, you will have a more accurate first touch.** Looking at the picture for reference, use Part B to take a moving first touch with the hardest part of your foot, which can be referred to as the "bat."

A moving first touch is not meant to push the ball far away from you; instead, it is intended for you to take the first step in the direction that you want to go. Implementing this one tip changed my soccer game and speed overnight. **A moving first touch will help your acceleration tremendously, because you will already start to build momentum and speed in the direction that you want to go, which will**

enable you to distance yourself from the defender who marks you.

To run faster, make sure that your arms travel from "eye socket" to "hip pocket;" unclench the body parts that do not help you run faster; sprint on the balls and toes of your feet, and practice sprinting to become faster. Finally, use a moving first touch in a soccer game to become a faster player immediately.

(Bonus Tip: If you are overweight, then losing some weight will help you become faster, because you will not have added mass slowing you down.)

If you are interested in learning more about how to correctly receive the ball to create more assists and score more goals, then grab a copy of the *Understand Soccer* series book, *Soccer Passing & Receiving*.

Chapter 2

How to Jump Higher with Plyometrics

Jump training, also known as plyometrics, is one of the most important areas of fitness that a soccer player can train. Plyometric training increases your rate of force development, explosiveness, and sprinting speed. More importantly, it increases acceleration speed, which is critical for a soccer player. **Being able to jump higher will not only help with your ability to head the ball but will also make you a more explosive and quicker runner.** Whether you prefer to have an entire jump training workout, have plyometrics as part of your warm-up, or add a few sets at the end of a workout to help your soccer game, jump training is one of the most important non-soccer specific exercises.

Athletes can perform power-based movements before strength training and conditioning. **Therefore, warm-ups are a good place to jump train as it can increase muscle and force output.** Use these exercises to increase your jumping:

1. Depth Jumps
2. Standing Jumps
3. Box Jumps
4. Broad Jumps
5. Split Lunge Jumps
6. Jump Knee Tucks

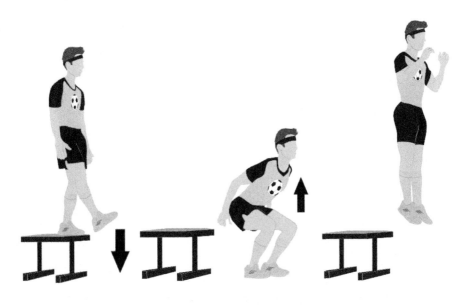

DEPTH JUMPS

1. **Depth jumps** involves stepping off a box/ledge/step, landing on the ground, and then jumping once your feet hit the ground. Depth jumps increase eccentric control and coordination of the hamstrings while allowing you to absorb more force safely. Land softly when stepping off the box. The depth jump is one of the best exercises an athlete can use to force overload. This technique is used by high jumpers, sprinters, and many basketball stars because of its effectiveness. Depth jumps strongly fatigue the central nervous system. Therefore, do not use these more than once per week, and do these first in a plyometric workout.

2. **Standing jumps** are simply jumping as high as you can while staying in one spot. Wait at least 20 seconds between each rep, because you are training for max jumping height. Think of it in terms of soccer; will you ever be repeatedly jumping up and heading the ball in a game? Or will you only need to jump as high as you can once to head the ball, with several minutes passing until you need to jump up to head the ball again?

3. **Box jumps** are when you jump up onto a box. Aim to use a box that is tall enough to challenge you, but not too tall that it will increase your chances of injury. Many gyms have wooden or metal boxes to train on, but anything sturdy and tall will work. A trick is to make sure that you engage your arms and use them to propel you onto the box. Many soccer players jump with only their legs. However, a proper jump is an explosive, full-body movement.

4. **Broad jumps** are when you stand flat-footed and with no momentum, jump forward as far as you can and land on both feet. These are great for generating raw jumping power because they are done with no momentum.

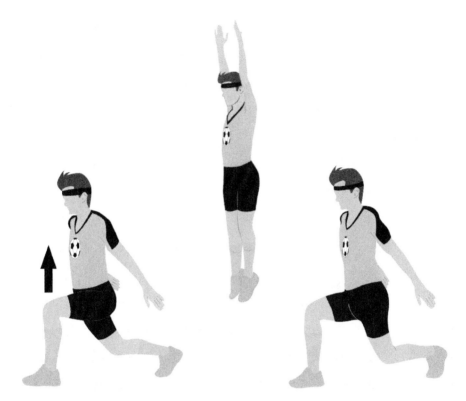

SPLIT LUNGE JUMP

5. **Split lunge jumps** start in a lunge position. Then, jump up and switch positions of your legs. If you started with a right-leg forward lunge, after one split lunge jump your left leg will be in front of you and your right leg behind you. This move is great for developing strength equally in each leg, with little involvement from the other leg during each jump. The other jumps in this chapter are done with both legs, so it is often hard to notice if one of your legs is weaker than the other. With this jump, you can see if there are any imbalances in strength in either leg, while really working your buttocks and hamstrings.

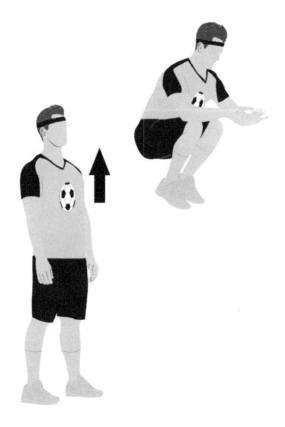

JUMP KNEE TUCKS

6. **Jump knee tucks** are a move done in one spot where you jump up and bring your knees as high as you can to tuck them into your chest. Jump knee tucks are also known as high knee jumps. These are great for working on your ability to get your feet quickly off the ground.

Plyometric (Jump Training) Workout

1. Depth Jumps - 3 sets, 1 rep each, rest 30 sec. between sets

2. Standing Jumps - 3 sets, 1 rep each, rest 30 sec. between sets

3. Box Jumps - 3 sets, 1 rep each, rest 30 sec. between sets

4. Broad Jumps - 3 sets, 1 rep each, rest 30 sec. between sets

5. Split Lunge Jumps - 2 sets, 4 reps each leg, rest 1 minute between sets

6. Jump Knee Tucks - 2 sets, 10 reps, rest 1 minute between sets

Notice that, until the last two jumps, you will do only one repetition per set. This is because you want to train in a way that will best carry over to your soccer performance. **Therefore, fewer reps with increased power are the best way to increase the height of your jumps, and the quickness of your sprints.**

Finally, notice that, for the duration of this entire workout, there are only 48 total repetitions. This is because you should care most about becoming more explosive and powerful. For years, I made the mistake of doing tons of repetitions in my plyometric workouts, which helped my muscular endurance but only added a few inches to the height of my jumps. Instead, I should have followed one of my high-school teammate's plyometric workouts, which looked like the workout in this chapter. During our senior year, he was only 5'5", but he could jump higher in the air and he won more headers than our 6'7" center back. Yes, you read that correctly; he out-jumped a player with a 14-inch height advantage!

YouTube: If you would like to do a jump training workout while receiving instruction from me, then watch the *Understand Soccer* YouTube video: *Soccer Conditioning Workouts at Home*.

Chapter 3

Should You Go for a Run?

Players, parents, and coaches often think that because games involve a lot of running, and there are no timeouts other than half-time, soccer players need to run long distances to be physically fit for a game. However, when analyzing most players, they jog or run only 70% of the actual game-time minutes. Most of those runs are explosive, high-intensity sprints, rather than long, slow jogs.

Jonas Forsberg researched many soccer games and said that soccer is a "power-sport," in which sprinting, maximum strength, and jumping are important. He mentioned that running long distances will not help players as much, because it will make them weaker and their sprinting slower. **Running long distances will build slow-twitch muscle fibers at the expense of fast-twitch muscle fibers, which are more important for soccer players.**

Therefore, soccer players should increase their conditioning by using dynamic sprinting drills, or high-intensity interval training (HIIT), such as:

Shuttle Sprints (Suicide Sprints) – Set cones down every five yards for 15 yards. Sprint to the first cone five yards away, and then back to the start. Next, sprint to the second cone 10 yards away, and then back to the start. Finally, sprint to the third cone 15 yards away, and then back to the start. Complete four total sets of this drill.

10-Yard Backward Sprints – Set cones down 10 yards apart and sprint backwards 10 yards. Rest 20 seconds between sprints. Complete eight total sets of this drill.

The only time that players should continuously run 1-2 miles is if they are being evaluated on them. This often happens in a tryout.

If you are interested in learning tips and tricks to double your chances of making a soccer team by having an amazing tryout, then grab a copy of the *Understand Soccer* series book, *Soccer Tryouts*.

Another long-distance sprint to be aware of is the "beep test," which is a favorite of some coaches. Coaches use the "beep test," (also known as the "multi-stage fitness test," "shuttle run test," or "PACER test") to judge a player's fitness. **The "beep test" involves running continuously between two spots that are 22 yards apart.** These runs are done with a prerecorded audio tape, which beeps at set intervals. As the test progresses, the interval between each successive beep reduces, thereby forcing the athlete to increase their speed over the course of the test, until they cannot stay coordinated with the recording.

This test has 23 levels, each of which lasts 60 seconds. There are several beeps at each 60-second level. The highest level that a soccer player can reach before failing is their score. Avoid running too fast in the beginning because you will tire out too quickly. Set your running pace to coordinate with the beeps; this will preserve your energy.

One of the best ways to perform well during this drill is to practice it. If you know that the coach will evaluate you on it, then find a "beep test" recording on YouTube and practice it on a field that is like the one on which you will be evaluated.

The highest documented score is Level 17, but fit male soccer players achieve a Level 13 and above, and fit female soccer players achieve a Level 12 and above.

Beep Test Scoring	Men	Women
Excellent	13+	12+
Very Good	11-12	10-11
Good	9-10	8-9
Okay	7-8	6-7
Bad	5-6	4-5
Very Bad	<5	<4

In conclusion, avoid doing cardio sessions by running continuously, unless you are going to be evaluated on it in a tryout. Otherwise, focus on more soccer-specific running drills (e.g., shuttle sprints) to work on your explosiveness and speed, which will directly transfer to the soccer field.

Chapter 4

High-Intensity Interval Training (HIIT)

For a cardiovascular exercise that will help your performance the most and will help you shed fat, consider High-Intensity Interval Training (HIIT). **HIIT is the process of alternating short periods of intense exercise with recovery periods.** These intense workouts usually last under 30 minutes. Soccer is a great example of HIIT training (i.e., walking then sprinting, walking then jogging, walking then sprinting again).

In Adam Bornstein's interview with soccer superstar David Beckham, he uncovered what David Beckham did during his career to improve his fitness on the soccer field. **Sure enough, David Beckham used High-Intensity Interval Training to stay in peak physical shape.** To perform any of Beckham's challenges listed in this chapter, you must first determine your maximum heartrate (MHR) using the following equation:

220 – (your age) = MHR

The percentages in these challenges refer to your maximum heartrate (MHR). Use a chest-strap heartrate monitor or activity tracker (e.g., a Fitbit) to track your heartrate.

Each sequence is its own workout, and these David Beckham workouts are examples of quick and easy ways to become fitter for your soccer games. You can either add one to the end of your weight-training session or perform one by itself.

Challenge 1: Five-minute run at 80% of your MHR. Rest four minutes between sets. Repeat five total sets.

Challenge 2: Two-minute run at 95% of your max heartrate. Rest one minute between sets. Repeat eight total sets.

Challenge 3: 20-second sprint as fast as you can. Rest one minute between sets. Repeat 30 total sets.

Challenge 4: Run 120 yards in 20 seconds. Rest 100 seconds between sets. Repeat 10 total sets.

Challenge 5: Sprint 60 yards. Rest 10 seconds between sets. Repeat eight total sets.

In conclusion, you can follow one of David Beckham's challenges or you can use other HIIT workouts to improve your cardiovascular endurance. **Also, HIIT can be done with other cardio exercises like biking, swimming, rowing, and jumping. Additionally, you can do HIIT with multi-joint weightlifting exercises too like deadlifts, squats, kettlebell swings, and dumbbell snatches.**

Chapter 5

Weight Loss

Have you ever struggled with losing weight? Have you ever felt like if you dropped a few pounds, then your confidence would go up? Well, this chapter will provide tips and things to avoid if you are interested in losing weight, as excerpted from the *Understand Soccer* series book, *Soccer Nutrition*. Even if you are not interested in losing weight, this chapter still has a ton of information that you may find interesting.

Here are some things to consider when trying to lose weight:

1. Know how many calories to eat in a day.
2. Find your ideal body fat percentage.
3. Get a Fitbit-
4. Drink more water.
5. Get enough sleep.
6. Do not cut out all fat.
7. Do not go low carb on soccer days.
8. Avoid thinking there is a magic pill.

First, when starting a weight-loss plan, it is important to understand what will happen when you stop the plan. Short-term weight loss can be maintained if you keep doing what allowed you to lose weight in the first place. **However, permanent weight loss requires a lifestyle change to ensure that your habits will allow you to keep losing weight, and you will not gain it back.** Therefore, if you really dislike doing certain weight-loss activities, then you must find more manageable activities that you can see yourself doing for the rest of your life.

Also, be aware that competitive athletes will need to lose weight differently than the average person. A regular person can lose weight by fasting or cutting carbs, whereas soccer players need to have a weight-loss plan to ensure that they can still perform on the field by eating their allotted carbs strategically around physical activity.

Weight Loss = Baseline Calories + Exercise > Calories Consumed

Baseline calories are the number of calories that your body would burn if you just lay in bed all day and did not move. To determine the number of calories that you burn in a day, add the baseline calories to the amount of activity you did (e.g., walking, running, weightlifting, playing soccer, etc.) **You will lose weight by burning more calories than you eat.**

To make it easy on yourself, go to the following website and let their calculator tell you how many calories you need to consume to maintain your current weight and give you a breakdown of the macronutrients needed for a person of your bodyweight: https://www.active.com/fitness/calculators/calories

For example, at the time of writing this chapter, I am 6' tall and weigh 195 lbs. I have an active lifestyle. The website shows that it will take 3,400 calories to maintain my bodyweight. It also suggests a range of carbs, proteins, and fats to consume. Because I am always looking to add more muscle, I aim to eat at least one gram of protein for every pound I want to weigh.

Next, I let the amount of activity in a day determine the number of carbs that I will consume. On days when I am writing and publishing books or videos, I am less active. Therefore, I will consume less carbs, because I do not need as much energy. I also eat more fat, so I will stay full. Therefore, on inactive days, I will eat about 300 grams of carbs, and 120 grams of fat.

My Inactive Days

200g protein x 4 calories/g = 800 calories from protein

300g carbs x 4 calories/g = 1,200 calories from carbs

120g fat x 9 calories/g = 1,080 calories from fat

Total = 3,080 calories (I eat less on days I am not active)

My Active Days

200g protein x 4 calories/g = 800 calories from protein

475g carbs x 4 calories/g = 1,900 calories from carbs

100g fat x 9 calories/g = 900 calories from fat

Total = 3,600 calories (I eat more on days when I am highly active)

There are 3,500 calories in a pound. Therefore, if I want to lose weight, then I need to eat less than the 3,400 calories needed to maintain my weight. Generally, trying to lose a pound a week (i.e., a 500-calorie deficit each day) will allow you to achieve your goal weight without having to drop your calories and energy levels drastically. However, remember that if you go back to your old habits, then the weight will come back, too. **Therefore, avoid focusing only on breaking a bad habit. Instead, replace a bad habit with a good habit.** For example, if you get a sugar craving and have a bad habit of eating chocolate, then a better habit would be to eat dark chocolate, and a good habit would be to eat a piece of fruit.

Second, as a soccer player with muscle, do not worry so much about your Body Mass Index (BMI) because body fat is a better way to measure your health. Doctors, dieticians, and nutritionists often judge whether a person is overweight by their BMI, but this is a scale better used for people who do not exercise. BMI treats fat and muscle the same which is not too helpful for a soccer player who has muscle mass which the average person does not. A better guide is how your body looks in the mirror and your body fat percentage.

Using myself as an example, I have a BMI of 27 which would place me in the overweight category. However, I play soccer about two times per week right now and weightlift three to four times per week. I have visible abdominals and a low body fat percentage. Therefore, by using myself as an example, it is easy to see that the BMI scale is faulty for someone who exercises regularly and weight trains often. Still unconvinced? Well, the 6'2" Cristiano Ronaldo in peak condition at 188lbs is considered overweight too, which we both know is laughable. **Therefore, below is a Body Fat Rating Chart which applies to adults ages 18 and older, based on findings from the American College of Sports Medicine, the American Council on Exercise, and various other scientific studies:**

Body Fat Rating	Women	Men	Fitness Level
Risky - Low	<15%	<5%	Unsafe - See a Licensed Health Care Professional
Ultra Lean	15-18%	5-8%	Elite Athlete
Lean	19-22%	9-12%	Optimal Health and Longevity
Moderately Lean	23-30%	13-20%	Good Health
Excess Fat	31-40%	21-30%	Excessive Fat
Risk - High	>40%	>30%	Unsafe - See a Licensed Health Care Professional

Use the same website mentioned previously to determine your body fat by entering your weight, waist circumference, hips circumference, wrist circumference, and forearm circumference. Sure, there are more precise ways to measure than this method, but this will give you a great estimate of your current body fat percentage:

https://www.active.com/fitness/calculators/calories

Third, buy a Fitbit/step counter/activity tracker. The recommended minimum of steps to walk per day is 8,000, but a 10,000-12,000 minimum is better if you are trying to lose weight. Walking burns the same number of calories as running; it just takes a little longer. **Walking enough steps per day is one of the most underrated ways to lose weight.** Think about it; soccer players take a lot of steps, which explains why they are often among the leanest athletes on the planet.

Fourth, drink more water to flush out toxins from your body and improve digestion. Drinking beverages with calories like juice, carbonated soda pop, and alcohol have "stealth calories." These calories come in mostly undetected by our bodies. **Scientific evidence confirms that although high-calorie beverages count towards our daily calories, the body does not detect them the same way as it would recognize solid food.** By consuming solid food, a person's body naturally compensates by reducing the rest of their food intake. However, when people ingest liquid calories, they do not compensate for them by eating fewer calories. This explains the results of a study by researchers from Harvard University and the Children's Hospital in Boston that found women who increased their intake of sugar-sweetened beverages, gained significantly more weight than those who did not.

Fifth, get enough quality sleep. Too little sleep means you will spend more hours in the day awake. More waking hours will result in eating more food, because your body is more likely to be hungry the longer you stay awake. More food means more calories, which makes it difficult to lose weight. **Furthermore, not getting enough sleep will increase the cortisol hormone in your body, which increases your appetite and stress levels.**

Sixth, do not cut all fat from your meal plan. **You need fat to use the fat-soluble vitamins A, D, E, & K properly. Also, fat helps with satiation—the feeling of fullness.** In an interview with *Men's Health Magazine*, nutritionist Jaime Mass, R.D. said, *"When you remove fat from a food product, it must be replaced with other ingredients to provide a tasty and profitable alternative. So, if you take a food with fat, remove it, triple the carbs, double the sugar, add extra ingredients to support the consistency and flavor, label it fat-free and consume it for years* *and years, you are setting yourself up to be overweight and develop health problems, including abdominal fat, Type 2 diabetes, and cardiovascular issues."*

Even worse, processed foods like low-fat ice cream and low-fat yogurt typically have more sugar and calories than their full-fat counterparts. Being fat-free is perfectly fine for foods like vegetables and most fruits because they are naturally fat-free. They do not need to be processed to remove fat. However, avoid picking fat-free versions of food that naturally has fat in it.

Seventh, avoid low-carb diets (e.g., the ketogenic diet). Low-carb diets are more reasonable for people who are not athletes, as they will need less energy from carbohydrates. However, soccer players need carbs to fuel their training and games. **If you must, then consider reducing your carb intake only on days when you will not play soccer.** Carbs you should cut are "white" carbs (e.g., white bread, white rice, white potatoes, white pasta, and white sugar). These and other refined grains are low in nutrients, while whole-grain bread, oatmeal, sweet potatoes, and brown rice are high in fiber and rich in B-vitamins.

Eighth, avoid thinking there is a "magic pill" which you can take that will do the work for you. Thinking there are magic pills is not good because you develop the habit of looking for the easy way out. Thinking there are "overnight successes" is just as problematic because you do not see the 10 or so years of hard work that person did to become successful. **Leave the mindset of finding a magic pill and becoming an overnight success to other people who wish everything were easier.** The trick is knowing that things rarely become easier, you simply become better.

In conclusion, remember the following pointers to ensure you do not fall into weight loss traps which so many other people do:

1. Determine how many calories you need in a day.
2. Aim for an ideal body fat percentage.
3. Invest in an activity tracker to count your steps.
4. Avoid drinks with calories.
5. Get enough sleep.
6. Avoid fat-free foods or a fat-free diet.
7. Eat plenty of carbs on days you train or play soccer.
8. Avoid looking for magic pills and overnight success.

Section on
Weight Training

Chapter 6

Why Weight Train as a Soccer Player?

As a soccer player, your focus of physical activity should be to improve your game. Assuming that you are training/practicing regularly and playing in competitive matches at least once per week, weight training is another activity to have an edge over your competition. **As beneficial as weight training is for a soccer player, do not place weight training above practice, training, or games, but use it to boost your on-the-field performances while you are away from the field.**

Personally, I made the mistake of thinking weight training was just as important as soccer training to become better at soccer. This mindset held me back because I would sometimes train my legs a day or two days before a game and would be so fatigued that I could hardly run in the warm-up prior to the start of the game. Make sure your soccer priorities are to maximize weight training's benefit on your ability to play soccer.

First, a reason to weight train is that a pound of fat is three times larger than a pound of muscle. Therefore, by weight training, you will become leaner and fitter for soccer. If you are a female, then do not worry that weight training will "bulk" you up, because even if you gain a few pounds, you will still lose several inches in many areas of your body, thereby making you appear much leaner. Afterall, a pound of fat is three times larger than a pound of muscle. **Additionally, a pound of muscle burns up to 50 calories per day, while a pound of fat burns only five calories per day.** More muscle mass will make it easier for your body to use calories as fuel, instead of storing them as fat. Furthermore, weight training will help you in soccer by improving your speed, strength, muscular endurance, and body fat.

Also, weight training will make it tougher for your opponents to push you off the ball, give you harder shots, and allow you to jump higher when going up for a header. All these things will help you create more assists, score more goals, help your team dominate games, and build your confidence.

Second, not only will weight training help you build soccer confidence (i.e., your confidence as a soccer player on the field), but it will also boost your confidence in everyday life. Just think about the confidence boost that you will get from looking great at the beach, having six-pack abdominal muscles on the soccer field, or showing off the definition in your arms and legs in your everyday outfits. **Having a better physical appearance will make it easier to believe in yourself and achieve more.**

Third, weight training will build discipline that will transfer to other areas of your life. This is because weight training can function as a "keystone habit" in your life. According to Charles Duhigg's book, *The Power of Habit*, keystone habits are: "*Small changes that people introduce into their routines that unintentionally carry over into other aspects of their lives.*" **When it comes to weight training and exercise in general, studies show that people who exercise three or more times per week eat healthier, consume fewer alcoholic beverages, smoke less, have more productive days, and sleep better than people who do not exercise regularly.**

Finally, if you decide to weight train, and you have games and practices that occur in the same week, then consider only weightlifting two times per week. In the offseason, when you are practicing soccer 1-2 times per week, consider working on plyometric jump training, and you can weight train even more than twice a week if you want to. Since you will have fewer soccer games and practices, your body will have more time to recover from weight training workouts.

The benefits of weight training are noticeable on the field; you will become faster, more explosive, and more agile. Also, your improved physical appearance will have the added benefit of boosting your confidence. Therefore, as a soccer player, it is recommended that you weight train at least twice per week. Consider one upper-body workout and one lower-body workout to develop a balanced physique.

Chapter 7

Big Lifts to Increase Performance

As a soccer player interested in understanding the benefits of weight training, it is important that you "train movements, not muscles." Also, it is key to work muscles equally to avoid imbalances that can lead to sprains, strains, and tears. For example, not only does balance mean doing as many dumbbell chest presses with your right arm as with your left, but it also means that you are training push and pull muscles equally. Therefore, for every chest workout you perform, there should be a back workout planned, too. Similarly, if you have a "pushing" leg exercises like squats or leg presses, you should also have a "pulling" leg exercise like deadlifts and Romanian deadlifts.

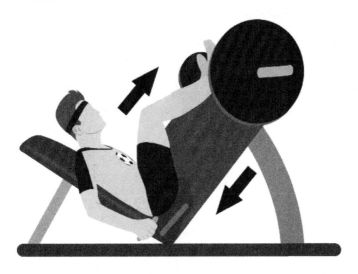

LEG PRESS

When weight training, perform the movements that will help you most as a soccer player. Squatting is more important than bicep curls, just as deadlifting is more important than triceps extensions. **When you select a workout routine, it is important to prioritize what are called "multi-joint/compound movements" (e.g., squats, deadlifts, rows, bench presses, and overhead presses), instead of "single-joint/isolation movements" (e.g., leg extensions, leg curls, chest flyes, bicep curls, and triceps extensions).** Similarly, training in plyometric movements (e.g., jumping off one foot and vertical jumps) are important, too. These are covered in the speed and endurance section of this book.

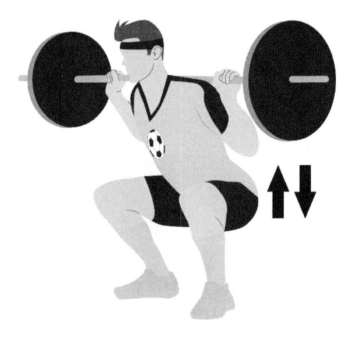

SQUAT

When doing any exercise, it is important to understand how many repetitions you will need to perform. **For example, when doing a set of squats, each time you squat down and stand back up is one repetition.** Therefore, a "set" is made up of the repetitions you do without stopping.

Soccer players walk plenty of steps and perform a lot of physical activity just by playing soccer. This means they should perform an appropriate number of sets (and repetitions in each set) to maximize their performance, while minimizing their time spent in the gym.

Here are the three general rep ranges for a set:

1. 6 or less reps - strength
2. 8-12 reps - muscle size
3. 14+ reps - muscular endurance

*(**Note:** Your legs, calves, and abdominal muscles will benefit from slightly higher reps per set than described in the above list. Also, the rep range listed assumes that you will finish your last repetition of a set without being able to do another repetition with good form. **When lifting, it is important that you work until failure. This will help your muscles grow faster.**)*

So, the above list may lead you to the question, "How many reps should I do in each set?" Well, regularly playing in soccer games that last 45-90 minutes will result in a considerable amount of muscular endurance in your legs already. If you play in the midfield and are expected to do a lot of running, then training for muscular endurance in the 14+ rep range can be helpful. The 8-12 rep range leads to hypertrophy, which is also known as "muscle size." For example, 250-pound bodybuilders who are tremendously ripped and have large muscles train in the 8-12 rep range. Gaining muscle may seem impressive and build your confidence, but large muscles should not be a soccer player's highest priority, because they may slow you down. **Therefore, the most ideal rep range for a soccer player is six or fewer reps, assuming you have access to a gym. If not, then going to failure, is what you should focus on.**

Remember the Individual Soccer Player's Pyramid in the preface of this book; it shows you how fitness is less important to train than the technical skills of soccer like passing, shooting, foot skills, and defending. Therefore, more time should be spent on those and less on weight training. This means that we need to get the most out of our time in the gym. Because playing soccer involves so much running, growing big muscles will slow us down, and training for muscular endurance will use up a lot of our calories that we will need to increase the strength of our muscles by rebuilding them after we break them down. Furthermore, understand that quick and jerky reps are not good for long-term physical wellness. **As a soccer player, you are already susceptible to injury, so have controlled movements when weight training to limit any injuries.**

Also, having stronger muscles will allow you to sprint faster, jump higher, and kick the ball harder. These are all important skills for a soccer player to have because being good at soccer is highly related to being explosive. **Want to know the secret behind why so many of Lionel Messi and Cristiano Ronaldo's foot skills work? It is because they push the ball and sprint explosively away from the defender after they perform a skill.** Therefore, the more strength your muscles can use to explode, the quicker you will travel past the defender to create an assist or score for your team. If you are interested in learning about the foot skills that make Messi and Ronaldo so good, then grab a copy of the *Understand Soccer* series book, *Soccer Dribbling & Foot Skills*.

Now, understand that training in any of these rep ranges will still help the muscles in the other rep ranges, too. Doing a set of just five repetitions of squats will help you train primarily for strength, but you will still increase your muscle size and endurance, too. **Therefore, when weight training, go for strength and power if you want the largest impact on your** soccer performance. **Only 2-3 sets per exercise is needed to see an increase in strength.** Performing workouts with 12 sets and 4-6 exercises is good for a soccer player but performing workouts with 30 sets and 10-15 exercises is too much. Sadly, I made that mistake for years.

Additionally, according to the National Center for Health Research study led by sport psychologist C.I. Karageorghis, **listening to music can improve athletic performance in two ways: (1) by delaying fatigue, and (2) by increasing work capacity.** This study showed that listening to music leads to *"higher-than-expected levels of endurance, power, productivity, or strength."* To get the most out of music, listen to music with at least 140 beats per minute (BPM), such as upbeat rock-and-roll.

In summary, as a soccer player, you should train for movements, and not specific muscles. Also, listen to fast-paced music while training for an added boost. Use compound lifts of six or fewer repetitions to build strength quickly, such as:

Lower Body
-Squats
-Deadlifts
-Romanian Deadlifts
-Lunges
-Leg Presses
-Calf Raises (although not a compound lift)

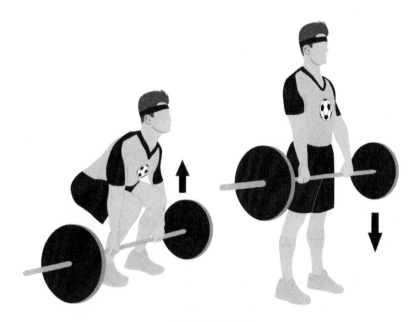

DEADLIFT

Upper Body

-Bench Presses
-Dips
-Overhead Presses
-Hip Huggers
-Rows
-Pull-Ups

Abdominals (Abs)*

-Ab Wheel
-Planks
-Sit-Ups
-Crunches
-Leg Raises

*Although many abs exercises are not compound lifts, they still bring stability to your core.

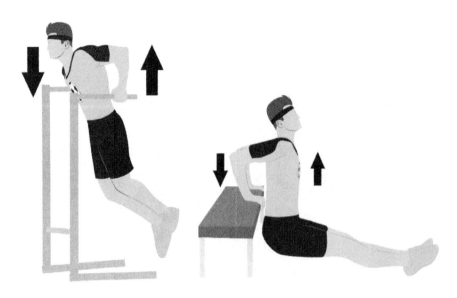

DIP   **BENCH DIP**

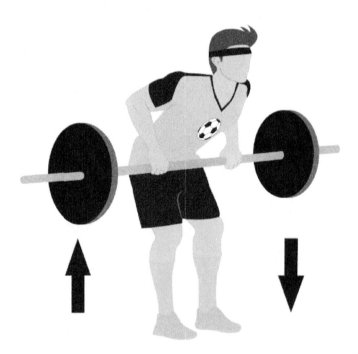

ROW

Chapter 9

Cristiano Ronaldo's Workout Plan

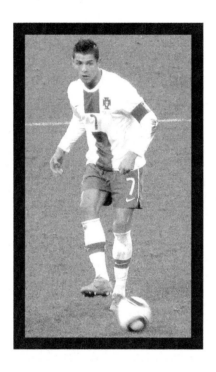

When considering the type of approach to take for weight training and conditioning in the gym, it is best to look at the players who are most admired for their on-field performances. Cristiano Ronaldo is one of the hardest workers the game has ever seen. He trains 3-4 hours per day, five days a week. Ronaldo has said, *"Pair all that with eight hours of sleep a night, and you're living strong in every sense of the concept."* Ronaldo realizes the importance of a full night's sleep to have enough energy to work out and perform at the top of his game.

(**Note:** *If you struggle with falling asleep and/or staying asleep, and you want to know the tricks to wake up feeling well rested every morning, then consider grabbing a copy of the Understand Soccer series book, Soccer Sleep.*)

Ronaldo is also an advocate of changing up his routines and never doing the same thing repeatedly, because he knows that the human body is quick to adapt to a workout.

Ronaldo emphasizes four major fitness areas:

1. Warm-Up
2. Soccer Practice
3. Conditioning
4. Weight Training

This chapter will cover his conditioning away from the soccer field and the weight training he does in the gym. He has a good deal of soccer-specific drills and conditioning exercises during his team's practice as well as he often stays after practice to work on his free kicks. The section of this book on *Stretching and Flexibility* has great tips for your warm-ups. **Cristiano Ronaldo knows it is just as important to train his mind because wherever the mind leads, the body follows. He says, "*Learn to train your mind as well as your body. Mental strength is just as important as physical strength and will help you achieve your goals.*"** Therefore, since this chapter is all about training the body, grab a copy of the *Understand Soccer* series book, *Soccer Mindset*, to learn how to train your mind. Now, let us dive into one of Cristiano Ronaldo's workout plans, per the article by Jacob Osborn on www.manofmany.com. Google/YouTube any exercises that are unfamiliar to you.

Warm-Up (no rest in between moves):

- Hip Twisters – 50 seconds
- Side-Lying Clams – 40 seconds each side
- Side-lying T-Stretch – 40 seconds each side
- Bird-Dogs – 50 seconds
- Bodyweight Squats – 50 seconds
- Reverse Lunges – 40 seconds

Fast Leg Workout (rest 20 seconds after the last move of each section):

Section 1:
- Single-Leg Glute Bridges – 40 seconds each leg
- Dumbbell Reverse Lunges – 30 seconds each leg
- Drop Squats – 40 seconds

Section 2:
- Side-Lying Leg Raises – 50 seconds each leg
- Dumbbell Walking Lunges – 50 seconds
- Jump Squats – 30 seconds

Section 3:
- Cross back Lunges – 40 seconds each leg
- Bulgarian Lunges – 40 seconds each leg
- Bodyweight Squats – 30 seconds
- Jump Squats – 30 seconds

Cristiano Ronaldo's Off-Season Gym Workout Plan:

Monday: Circuit Training
Do the following circuit three times:
- Barbell Squats – 8 reps
- Box Jumps – 10 reps
- Broad Jumps – 8 reps
- Split-Leg Jumping Lunges – 8 reps each leg
- Lateral Bounds – 10 reps

Tuesday: Rest

Wednesday: Circuit Training
Repeat the following circuit three times:
- Pull-Ups – 10-15 reps
- Bench Dips – 20 reps
- Push-Ups – 20-30 reps
- Medicine Ball Toss – 15 reps
- Push Press – 10 reps

Thursday: Quadriceps and Conditioning
- Power Cleans – 5 reps for 5 sets

- Sprints – 200 yards for 8 sets

Friday: Abdominals and Core
- One-Arm Side Deadlifts – 5 reps with each arm for 3 sets
- Dumbbell One-Legged Deadlifts – 10 reps for 2 sets
- Knee Tuck Jumps – 10-12 reps for 3 sets
- Overhead Slams – 10-12 reps for 3 sets
- One-Leg Barbell Squats – 5 reps for 2 sets
- Hanging Leg Raises – 10-15 reps for 3 sets

Saturday: Rest

Sunday: Conditioning
- Jumping Rope – 10 sets with 1 minute of rest between sets
- Resistance Sprinting – 50 yards for 10 sets

Ronaldo's workout intensity, frequency, exercises, and duration are always changing around his game schedule. It is not advisable to train your legs the day before a game. Use the workout plan in this chapter as a guideline for your workouts to understand the emphasis that top-level soccer players place on leg strength, speed, endurance, and power. Notice how Ronaldo trains his upper body much less than his lower body.

YouTube: If you would like to watch a video on one of Ronaldo's workout, then watch the *Understand Soccer* YouTube video: *Cristiano Ronaldo's Gym Workout*.

Chapter 10

Should You Weight Train Your Upper Body?

Ever wonder if you should be training your upper body to increase your performance on the soccer field? Individual muscles of each movement must do their job to function as a strong unit. If you are kicking a ball, taking a long throw-in, or sprinting, these all involve transfer of force through your upper body. Therefore, though not as important as training your legs, training your upper body will still help improve your soccer game. However, if you are still growing in height, consider only doing calisthenics and not using weights. Do movements like push-ups, pull-ups, bodyweight squats, and sit-ups.

Cristiano Ronaldo, Alex Morgan, and Zlatan Ibrahimović all train their upper bodies in addition to their legs to help with their on-the-field abilities. Not only will a chiseled physique give you more confidence, but a strong upper body will also improve lower body lifts too (e.g., your lats will fire more so you will be better at deadlifts).

For exercise selection, choose moves that are multi-joint/compound exercises, such as:

Chest, Shoulders, & Triceps

Push Ups
Bench Presses
Overhead Presses
Dips

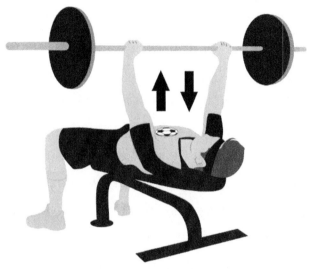

BENCH PRESS

Back, Biceps, & Traps

Pull-Ups
Pulldowns
Rows
Hip Huggers

Abdominals

Sit-Ups
Crunches
Planks
Leg Raises

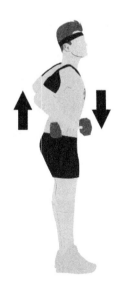

HIP HUGGERS

*(**Note:** Hip huggers are the opposite of dips. To do a dip, you will push weight down at your sides (i.e., push your body up with your arms at your sides). To do a hip hugger, you will pull weight up by your sides, just like if you were pulling your pants up. Do hip huggers and avoid upright rows. To do an upright row, you will pull weight in front of you, upwards towards your chin, while driving your elbows outwards. This is bad for your shoulders and will lead to pain if done for years.)*

Personally, I did not know very much about weightlifting initially. I started using the Beachbody workout program, P90X, so that I could work out alongside a professional trainer without having to pay the large fees to work with someone one-on-one. After I completed the 90-day P90X workout program multiple times, I also completed several other in-home video-training programs. They are good for general fitness if you do not want to pay a trainer. **Also, you will not need to create an exercise plan yourself, but can do it "alongside" others in the video, while the music that plays on the video will help improve your performance.**

In conclusion, upper body weight training will help you, but it should never be more important than soccer practice, games, or lower body training. Upper body weight training will surely help improve your confidence, increase your fitness, and help your abilities on the field.

Chapter 11

Weight Training Workout Template

As a soccer player whose focus is soccer, it is important to have a workout plan in place. Your weight training should revolve around practices and games, given that those are more important. Make sure to properly warm up, as directed in the chapter on how to warm up. During the off-season, consider weight training three times per week along with a couple of endurance, speed, or plyometric training sessions, too. Here is a weekly off-season weight training workout:

Weight Training - Off-Season

Monday - Upper Body Pull

Exercise	Sets	Reps
Pull-Ups	3	Max
Rows	3	5-6
Hip Huggers	3	5-6
*Dumbbell Curls	3	6-8
Leg Raises	3	Max

Wednesday - Lower Body

Exercise	Sets	Reps
Squats	3	5-6
Deadlifts	3	5-6
Lunges	3	6-8
Calf Raises	3	12-15
Planks	3	Max

Friday - Upper Body Push

Exercise	Sets	Reps
Bench Presses	3	5-6
Dips	3	Max
Overhead Presses	3	5-6
*Triceps Extensions	3	6-8
Sit-Ups	3	Max

*Optional exercise for a smaller body part.
Perform a warm-up that includes warm-up
sets of exercises above with reduced
Take sets to failure.

During the season where you have soccer games and practices 3-4 times per week, weight training is less important and should involve working the entire body to

avoid becoming too sore in any one specific area of your body. Here is a full-body in-season workout:

Weight Training - During Season		
1-2X per Week		
Exercise	**Sets**	**Reps**
Squat	2	5-6
Deadlift	2	5-6
Calf Raises	2	12-15
Bench Press	2	5-6
Pull-Ups	2	Max
Overhead Press	2	5-6
Rows	2	5-6
Sit-Ups	2	Max
Leg Raises	2	Max

Make sure to grab the free 1-page PDF printout with these off-season and in-season workouts to easily take them to your workout using the following link:

UnderstandSoccer.com/free-printout

Finally, here is a bodyweight only workout that can be performed at home or on the field. For any of the exercises listed that you are unfamiliar with, Google or YouTube them for a video demonstration.

Bodyweight Training - On-the-Field		
Exercise	Sets	Reps
Squat	2	Max
Lunges	2	Max
Calf Raises	2	Max
Push-Ups	2	Max
Back Widow	2	Max
Pike Presses	2	Max
Supermans	2	Max
Sit-Ups	2	Max
Planks	2	Max

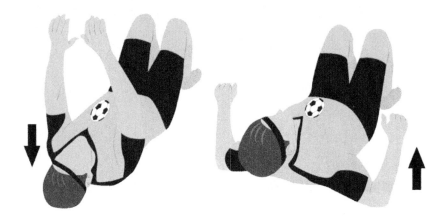

BACK WIDOW

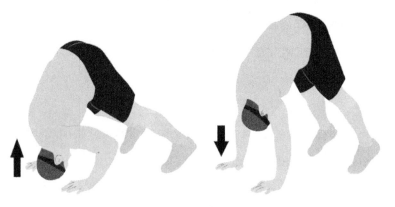

PIKE PRESS

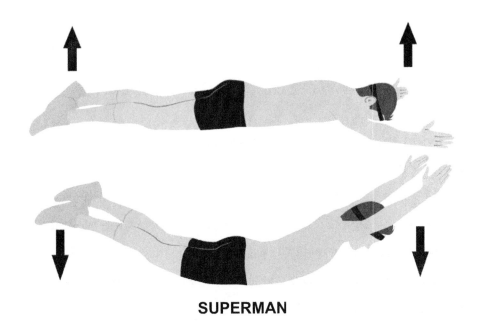

SUPERMAN

Finally, do not forget to cool down. With any cool-down, hold static stretches of the muscles you used in the workout. **One trick to reduce the time spent working out is once you are finished training a body part and move on to the next body part, you can use the time between each set to stretch the muscles that you just exercised.** For example, in the workout pictured, after the push-ups and pike presses, you can stretch your chest, shoulders, and triceps in between sets of the back exercises, back widow and supermans.

YouTube: If you would like to do the bodyweight training workout while receiving instruction from me, then watch the *Understand Soccer* YouTube video: *Soccer Strength Training at Home*.

Chapter 12

How to Eat to Gain Muscle

In the section of this book on speed and endurance, a chapter discussed how to lose weight. This chapter is for those under-sized soccer players who would improve their performance by gaining weight. Remember from the weight loss chapter that to lose weight, we must use more calories than we consume. Therefore, this chapter is all about learning how to eat more calories than we use in a day.

First, the single easiest thing to gaining more weight is to add another meal each day. If you only eat three meals, add another meal before bed that can easily provide you with another 400-500 calories. If eating sounds like too much work, then consider protein shakes instead. Although it is recommended to eat a full meal before bed involving things like a vegetable, dairy, seeds, and nuts, drinking a protein shake with milk is better than nothing if you are trying to gain muscle. If you are looking for a protein powder to add to your protein shake prior to bed, use casein protein. Casein protein is the slowest digesting protein and will help feed your muscles for up to seven hours overnight.

Second, eat more food near your weight training, running, practices, or games. Calories prior to exercise will help fuel you to perform better during physical activity. Calories immediately after exercise are more likely to help rebuild your muscles and help you gain weight. Therefore, make sure to always have a post-workout meal or protein shake to obtain those added calories.

Finally, it is important to not just eat anything in sight. **A pound gained from eating fast foods will differ from a pound gained from eating healthy foods.** The cleaner the calories, the more muscle will be added for each pound of weight gain. Eat unhealthy foods, and each pound gained will contain more fat. Remember that the goal is to gain weight by gaining muscle. Adding muscle mass will help you perform even better on the field. Adding fat to your frame will only slow you down.

In summary, to gain more weight, you will need to eat more. The best way to do this is by adding a meal each day. Then, see how much you weigh, how you look, and how you feel after a month to decide if you need to add more food to each meal or add another meal to each day to gain more size.

Chapter 13

Deload Weeks

A deload week is a week where you limit your training to enable your body to recover fully and come back stronger afterwards. Research on deload weeks reveals they help us better recover from our workouts. Training breaks down our muscles, which temporarily decreases areas of our fitness like our strength. As we recover by using deload weeks, the body adapts and becomes stronger for the next session which is known as supercompensation. Yes, deload weeks allow us to workout less and get more muscles and gains in the gym.

If you push yourself too hard at the gym and on the field for too long without recovery, then you can burn out and experience symptoms like joint aches, pains, fatigue, and reduced motivation to train. This creates a plateau, because as your gains level off, you will no longer see improvements in your strength. As a soccer player, you should schedule a deload week from weight training every 4-8 weeks, as it is difficult to take a week off during the middle of the soccer season, when you will still have practices and games.

When meal planning for a deload week, plan to eat at your maintenance calorie level. Avoid too much high-

intensity cardio, as the goal of a deload week is to reduce the stress placed on your body and central nervous system. During this week, use light-intensity activities instead, such as walking and stretching.

Even in the English Premier League—the top-flight of English soccer—they have just implemented a weekend off during their season. All English clubs are guaranteed a minimum of 13 days between games, which is the same as in Italy and Spain, because they better understand the importance of recovery and injury prevention for their players. If you are concerned that you do not have a week you can take off in the middle of the season, then consider finding 2-3 periods of 3-4 consecutive days during which you do not have games to allow yourself to refrain from any physical activity. If you must do something, then this is a great time to work on your stretching and mobility movements instead.

In summary, use deload weeks as follows:

1. Use a deload week every 4-8 weeks.
2. Eat your maintenance level of calories.
3. Use light activity (e.g., walking and extra stretching).

Section on Stretching and Flexibility

Chapter 14

Why Stretch?

Weight training, cardio, and playing soccer can often lead to muscle imbalances because of three major reasons:

1. Players often favor one foot over the other.
2. Athletes run using body mechanics that are hard on their joints.
3. People do not always perform weightlifting exercises with perfect form.

However, stretching helps reset the body to help reduce the chances of injury. **Muscles shorten and become tight without stretching. Therefore, when you use your muscles during physical activity, they will be stiff and have a short range of motion. If your muscles do not have a wide range of motion, then you are at risk for joint pain, strains, and muscular damage.**

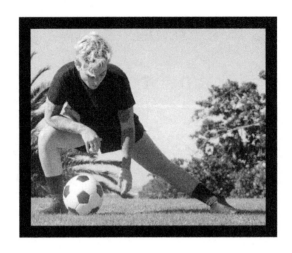

David Nolan, a physical therapist at Harvard-affiliated Massachusetts General Hospital says do not worry about stretching every muscle in your body, as this would take a long time. **He says, "*The areas critical for mobility are in your lower extremities: your calves, your hamstrings, your hip flexors in the pelvis and quadriceps in the front of the thigh. Stretching your shoulders, neck, and lower back is also beneficial.*"**

Remember that stretching takes time to reveal its benefits, just like eating nutritious foods takes time to become healthy, and weight training takes time to build muscle. **Consistency is key.** Therefore, make sure that you stretch before and after exercise. Also, when you are just relaxing and watching television, this is a great time to stretch, foam roll, or use a percussion/massage gun on your muscles, too.

A fun and quick test that you can do right now to reveal the importance of flexibility is to:

1. Stand up and point your feet diagonally away from you and attempt to squeeze your buttocks as hard as you can.
2. See how hard you can squeeze.
3. Next, while standing, point your feet inwards towards each other and try to squeeze your buttocks as hard as you can.
4. Notice that you can barely squeeze your buttocks at all.

After completing the example, it will be easier to understand that poor flexibility in different areas of your body can really affect your body's ability to generate power and force. This means that you cannot jump as high, run as fast, or kick a ball as hard as you could if you were more flexible. Therefore, stretch during your free time, as well as before and after games, to ensure that limited mobility does not prevent you from performing your best and does not result in an injury.

Chapter 15

Static vs Ballistic vs Dynamic Stretching

There are several ways you can stretch. One type of stretching is best to do before exercise, another way is best to do after exercise is completed, and yet another way should be avoided altogether. Let us dive into the three general types of stretching.

First, many people often confuse dynamic and ballistic stretching. In fact, I thought they were the same thing for many years without ever realizing one is recommended prior to exercise, and the other should be avoided. **Dynamic stretching is a controlled and coordinated stretch with a defined range of motion. Ballistic stretching is uncontrolled, uncoordinated, and usually involves momentum and bouncing.** Use dynamic stretching as a warm-up prior to a sports activity to push blood to the muscle and synovial fluids (lubrication) into the joints.

For years, the fitness industry promoted ballistic stretching. Prior to the most up-to-date understanding of exercise kinesiology, many fitness organizations and trainers believed bouncing lower at the end of each stretch by using momentum to create even more elasticity in the muscles was good. **Sadly, these jerky movements increase your risk of injuring muscles.** When using momentum to bounce beyond the normal elasticity in your muscles, you can tear muscle and damage soft tissues, according to the America Sports & Fitness Association (ASFA).

Finally, static stretches are held in a mildly uncomfortable position for usually between 20-60 seconds. **Static stretching is the most common form of stretching found in fitness. It is safe and effective to improve overall flexibility.** Static stretching is best when done after practice, games, training, or weightlifting.

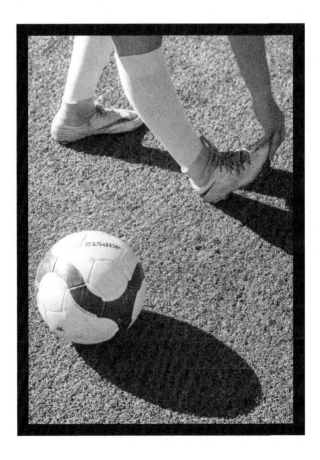

In summary, here are the three different types of general stretching:

1. Ballistic Stretches (avoid)—Stretches using bouncing. An example is bouncing at the bottom of a bent over hamstring stretch to travel a bit deeper in the stretch.

2. Dynamic Stretches (do <u>before</u> exercise)—Movement based stretches and warm-ups to improve performance and reduce the chance of injury. Examples include leg swings, trunk rotations, and arm rotations to "loosen" up the joints and muscles.

3. Static Stretches (do <u>after</u> exercise)—Hold a stretch for 20-60 seconds to promote recovery and increase flexibility. An example is holding a bent-over hamstring stretch, in which you try to touch your toes without bouncing, then with each exhale, you go deeper into the stretch.

Chapter 16

How to Warm Up Before Physical Activity

A warm-up is the time spent prior to your practice or game where you are "warming" your body up. The movement that you want to do depends on the activity you will be doing. **Usually, a warm-up will consist of light cardiovascular exercises combined with dynamic stretches.** Examples of dynamic stretches and light cardiovascular exercises are where you are shaking your arms/legs out, performing jumping jacks, doing standing mountain climbers, jogging, and performing short distance sprints. The two most important reasons to warm up the body before practicing or playing in a game is to prepare your body to be ready right when the game starts and to help prevent injury.

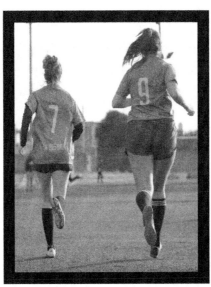

Incorporating cardiovascular exercises into your warmup will increase blood circulation, push synovial fluids into your joints, increase your body temperature, and boost your heartrate to prepare your body for more difficult activities.

Dynamic stretching warms your muscles and prepares you for the movements that you must conduct during physical activity. Your intensity should increase as you progress through your warmup to get closer to the level of intensity that your body will experience during a practice or game.

Just as important as making sure your body is ready to perform at the start of a match, warming up your body also helps to prevent injury. **Warm muscles help prevent acute injuries such as hamstring strains. Also, warming up will prevent overuse injuries by allowing your body to prepare steadily and safely.** Substitutes in a game should also continue to jog and do dynamic stretches while they are waiting to join a game.

Since the aim of a warmup is to ready your muscles for peak performance during physical activity, **it is crucial that you do not hold any stretches/poses for longer than a couple of seconds because doing so will decrease your power output during athletic activity by up to 10%.**

Additionally, a study by the *Journal of Strength & Conditioning Research* showed that well-trained runners who performed static stretches before a one-mile run were on average 13 seconds slower than those who did not perform static stretches. This is because stretched muscles require more energy from your body to produce the same amount of force. Therefore, if you perform static stretches before a game (e.g., bending down to touch your toes for 30 seconds, pulling your foot behind your body to stretch your quadriceps for 30 seconds, or holding a calf stretch for 30 seconds), then you will only reduce your performance.

In addition to the light cardiovascular movements mentioned earlier in this chapter, it is also good that you focus on some soccer-specific moves to ensure your body is warmed up. Start with the progression of passing a ball, then softly shooting a shot, and then striking the ball with full power for a few repetitions too. **Any warm-up you do, you want to start with the easiest form of that movement and then build your way up to the harder and more game-like versions. You never want to start with sprinting for the beginning of your warm-up.** It is better to have a nice and easy walk that turns into a jog that then becomes a few 5-yard sprints.

So, how long should you warm up prior to a game or practice? **You should warm up for at least 15 minutes. The older you get, the more prone you are to injury, so you will want to warm up for even longer once you get past your teenage years.**

Do this 15-minute soccer warm-up prior to your next practice or game:

1. Juggle the ball—2 minutes
2. Light jog—1 minute
3. Medium paced jog—1 minute
4. Short distance 5-yard sprints—do 6 in 1 minute
5. Jumping Jacks—1 minute
6. Pass the ball with a wall or teammate—2 minutes
7. Cross the ball to a teammate—2 minutes
8. Shoot into a net with a rolling ball—2 minutes
9. Do a body feint (i.e., jab step) and then shoot—2 minutes
10. Self-passes (i.e., Iniesta or an "L")—1 minute

Should you want to learn more about two of the three most important skills, the self-pass and body feint, and to know when to use them in a game, grab the *Understand Soccer* series book, *Soccer Dribbling & Foot Skills*. **Most athletes, especially early in their career, avoid stretching or warming up because it just does not seem like it contributes that much. This mindset and lack of action is a very near-sighted way to look at your overall game. It is unnecessary to spend 45 minutes warming up before a game.** However, you should take at least 15 minutes before you will begin playing in a game.

Similarly, before you play a game or have a practice, you also want to perform the dynamic stretching before any weight training. **Especially with weight training, it is important that you warm up the muscles that you will be weight training.** You do not need to warm up your calves if you are performing a back workout. Similarly, you should never start with your maximum bench press weight on the bar. You want to start with just the bar. Then, increasingly add more weight after each warm-up set until your body, your joints, and your muscles feel ready to engage fully in that exercise. The few minutes to warm up before exercising are important to make sure that your body stays fit and healthy while performing at its highest level.

Do this 10-minute warm-up prior to your weight training workout:

1. Light jog in place—2 minute
2. High knees jogging—1 minute
3. Jumping jacks—1 minute
4. Butt-kick jogging in place—1 minute
5. Leg swings forward and backwards—10 reps each leg
6. Leg swings side-to-side—10 reps each leg
7. While swing your arms, give yourself body hugs—30 seconds
8. Shake out your arms—30 seconds
9. Do the first weight training move of your workout with a reduced weight—2 sets

YouTube: If you would like to watch a video on how to stretch before a game, then watch the *Understand Soccer* YouTube video: *Stretching Before a Soccer Game*.

Chapter 17

Warm Up Your Mind

It is important for a soccer player to warm up their body before a game. However, most soccer players forget that they should also warm up their minds. You can have a fully warmed-up body, but if your mind is not prepared to play, then you will find your performance lacking. Therefore, consider the following keys to a great pre-game mind warm-up, taken from the *Understand Soccer* series book, *Soccer Mindset*:

1. Have a Routine
2. Focus on Process Behaviors
3. Mentally Rehearse

Key #1: Have a Routine

A pre-game routine will ensure that you have a consistent plan to help you before a game and increase your internal locus of control. Pre-game routines consist of drills and dynamic stretches that push blood into the muscles and synovial fluids into the joints. *(**Note:** If you are a coach who wants some terrific, soccer-specific drills to use for your team, then grab a copy of the Understand Soccer series book, Soccer Drills.)*

Your pre-game routine should also focus on the mental side of your game. A routine is like a funnel that channels your focus to ensure that you are ready to play soccer. Pre-game routines will help you stay focused on the important items, while avoiding mental distractions.

For example, you should have a few phrases to tell yourself before every game, such as:

- I am calm, cool, and collected.
- I am a goal-scorer.
- I am a hard worker.
- I am prepared for this moment.
- I am focused.
- I am unstoppable.
- I am relentless.
- I am unshakable.
- I am a leader.
- I am a winner.

Key #2: Focus on Process Behaviors

Next, remember that soccer is a team sport with 22 players in total. Referees also help to decide the outcome of the game. Therefore, be focused on what you can control. **"Process behaviors" represent what a soccer player has** control over and can perform regardless of how the game is unfolding. **Things like being aggressive, playing hard, staying level-headed, keeping your head up, having fun, communicating, and being positive with yourself and teammates are examples of "process behaviors."** A soccer player can stay committed to these attitudes throughout a game, whether or not it is going well. Focus on the process, and you will increase the likelihood of positive results happening.

Key #3: Mental Rehearsal

Think about the things you can do in the game to make sure you perform most effectively. Given that I play as a striker for my team, some things I mentally rehearse and visualize before games are:

✓ Keeping my head down to keep my form together while shooting;
✓ Swiveling my head so that I know where the opposition is when I receive a pass from a defender or midfielder; and
✓ Using a self-pass when a defender reaches in for the ball.

Mental Routine + Physical Routine = Success

In conclusion, soccer is as much a mental game as it is a physical one. Focus on both your mental and your physical routines prior to game time to ensure your mind and body are ready to go. Understand that process behaviors are things you can always control because they help describe your mindset.

Additionally, mentally rehearse the items which you know will make the biggest impact on your game. These rehearsals are position-specific and should differ for each player. Finally, remember that you can also have a morning routine upon waking to start off your day right and ensure your eventual success.

Chapter 18

How to Cool Down

Just as warming up before a practice or game will reduce your chances of injury, so too will cooling down after you are done with the training or a match. Also, cooling down will help to jump-start your recovery process and reduce the soreness you feel the next few days. When cooling down, it is important that you do different stretches than the dynamic stretches and movements you perform before a game or practice.

After a game, practice, or other athletic performance, you should perform static stretches. At this point, your body is fatigued and very warm, therefore you should work on your flexibility by holding stretches for 20-60 seconds each. You should no longer be worried about power output anymore because you have already completed your training or match. Now is the time to focus on going deep into the stretches that will improve the longevity of your joints, as well as increase your muscle length, which will allow you to feel better, recover faster, and play the sport you love for longer.

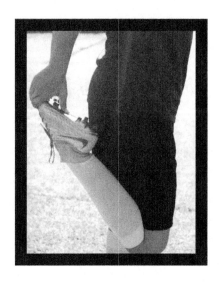

To cool down, pick a few basic stretches to perform for your hamstrings, quadriceps, glutes, hip flexors, adductors, abductors, and calves. Perform at least one stretch for each of those muscles to create a routine/habit that you can perform after every single practice or game. After the first several times stretching, the habit will stick, and you will hardly have to think about it before doing it. Remember that creating good habits will create a better you!

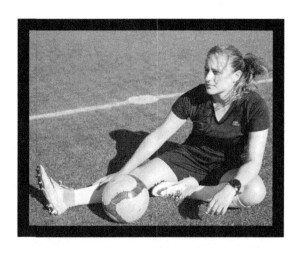

To stretch a muscle, pull or push it in the opposite direction in which you use it. For example, your hamstring muscle's major function is to pull your foot towards your buttocks. Therefore, to stretch your hamstrings, instead of moving your feet backwards towards your behind, move your feet forward to increase the distance between your feet and buttocks.

Use the following movements to stretch all the leg muscles that you engage when playing soccer:

- Using one or both arms while standing, pull one foot behind your body (to where you are bending at the knee). This will stretch your quadriceps (i.e., the muscles along the front of your thighs).

- While standing, place one ankle over your opposite knee and push on the knee of your bent leg to stretch your gluteus (i.e., your buttocks) and your abductors (i.e., the muscles along the outside of your thighs).

- Keeping both feet on the ground and reaching down (bending to touch your toes) will stretch your hamstrings (i.e., the muscles along the back of your thighs).

- Sitting on the ground and pulling your ankles between your legs while bending at the knees and pushing your elbows against your knees will stretch your adductors (i.e., the muscles along the inside of your thighs).

- Go into a lunge and place the knee of your back leg on the ground while driving your hips towards the floor. Using your arms to push against the knee in front of you, push your upper body backward and stretch out your hip flexor (i.e., the muscles atop the front of your thighs, where your hips are).

- In a plank position, drive your hips backward. This is like going into a downward dog pose, but only on the balls of your feet. Now, place one ankle on top of the other. Push yourself towards the space behind you to stretch your calves (i.e., the muscles that run along the back of your legs, below your knees).

For a soccer game or practice, you will use your leg muscles while running, dribbling, and kicking the ball. After a weight-training workout, you should cool down by stretching the muscle groups that you just used during your workout. Stretching your calves is not as helpful after a push-up and bench-press workout as stretching your chest. **Remember that the best time to use static stretches is after physical activity. Hold your stretches for 20-60 seconds each. Make sure that you take large inhales and exhales while holding each stretch. With each exhale, attempt to go deeper into the stretch, up to the point at which you are still slightly uncomfortable.**

Chapter 19

Other Options for Flexibility and Recovery

In this chapter, we will discuss many other ways to recover more quickly and improve your flexibility. With all forms of recovery, consistency is key, so do not expect any of these to rid you of your aches and pains after doing it only once. It usually takes years to break your body down. Therefore, it will at least take several months to build your body back up.

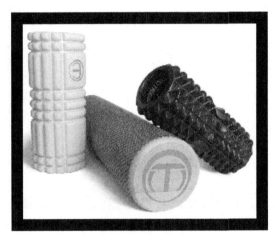

FOAM ROLLING

Foam rolling is often performed with a foam cylinder that you roll your body over to release muscle tension. Some people prefer using rolling pins over a foam roller, but they both serve the same purpose. Foam rolling is a form of self-massage that is often preferred by people who need a less-expensive option than massages or chiropractors. According to Michael Clark, Ph.D., physical therapist and CEO of the National Academy of Sports Medicine, *"Foam rollers can be a great part of a warmup or cooldown."* **Foam rolling improves circulation and prepares your muscles to stretch because rolling breaks down knots that limit your range of motion.**

When foam rolling, roll slowly. When you find a tender spot, focus in on it, until you feel it soften or release.

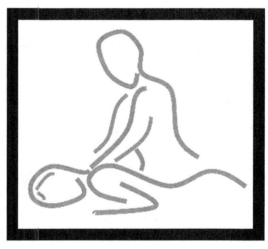

MASSAGE

A massage is a general term used for when someone presses or rubs your skin, muscles, tendons, and ligaments. Massages range from light pressure to deep pressure, depending on which massage you select. These are the most common types for a soccer player:

1. Swedish Massage–A gentle massage using long strokes, kneading, and circular movements for recovery and to relax.

2. Deep Massage–A more forceful massage using slower strokes to reach deeper layers of muscle and connective tissue. People with muscle damage from injuries usually prefer these massages.

3. Sports Massage–This form of massage is geared toward people involved in sport activities to help treat injuries. Usually, the injured area of the body receives all the attention.

4. Trigger Point Massage–This massage focuses on areas of tight muscle fibers from overuse or injuries.

According to the Mayo Clinic, massage is considered part of integrative medicine. It is increasingly being offered as treatment for a wide range of medical conditions while studies of the benefits of massage show that it is an effective treatment for reducing stress, pain, and muscle tension. Massage has been found helpful with:

- Anxiety
- Digestion
- Muscle pain and tenderness
- Headaches
- Insomnia caused by stress
- Soft tissue injuries
- Sports injuries
- Joint pain

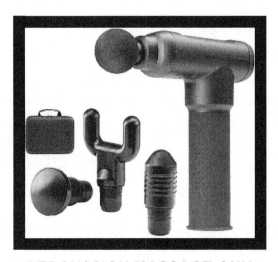

PERCUSSION MASSAGE GUN

Personally, I have found that foam rolling is inexpensive but takes a decent amount of movement on my part, as well as awkward positions to massage my muscles. I am less likely to do it than other forms of recovery because it requires me to be active, while I can use other options more passively. I have also found that I enjoy massages more because I can passively have someone massage me, but professional massages are expensive. Therefore, a great happy medium is a percussion massage gun. They range in cost from $60-$200, but you can get a decent one for $80. Therefore, this is more expensive than a foam roller but considerably less expensive than several professional massages. It is also semi-passive because you only need to put the head of the gun on the affected body part, and it does the work for you. The gun also comes with several attachments for different types of pressure.

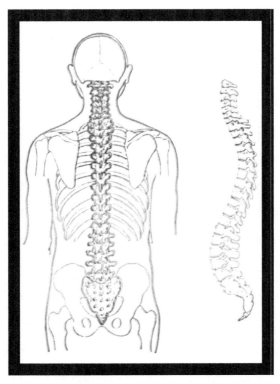

CHIROPRACTICE CARE

A chiropractor is a health care professional focused on the diagnosis and treatment of disorders using manual adjustment and manipulation of the spine. Chiropractors help reduce pain and improve performance. Many Major League Soccer (MLS) teams like the LA Galaxy and New York Cosmos treat back pain and other bodily injuries using chiropractic care. Chiropractors focus on the relationship between the nervous system and spine. They believe that a mis-aligned spine can affect the nervous system. For many conditions, chiropractic treatment can restore the structural integrity of the spine, reduce pressure on the sensitive neurological tissue, and consequently improve the health of the individual.

Personally, I have seen four different chiropractors for several months each. **The only type of chiropractor who has given me lasting relief for nagging injuries is a biophysics chiropractor, who used proven chiropractic techniques that corrected and restored my spine's alignment to ease pain from the source.** Two of the other three chiropractors only adjusted my spine when I was in pain, and the fourth one did little, while charging me a lot! Therefore, some chiropractors are well worth their cost, but many others are not, so if you decide to use a chiropractor to help reduce pain and improve recovery, then I recommend trying several different chiropractors and immediately finding a new one if your current chiropractor does not help you achieve results after a few visits.

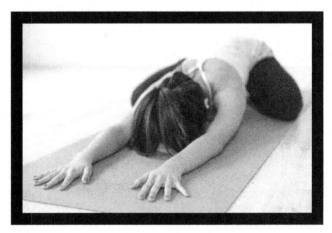

YOGA

Yoga is a mind and body practice with a 5,000-year history in ancient Indian philosophy. Various styles of yoga combine physical postures, breathing techniques, and meditation. Personally, I do not subscribe to any of the spiritual teaching related to yoga, but I have performed many of the stretches and poses associated with it. Honestly, yoga will help you with being flexible and to relax, but some of the poses are not soccer specific. The moves and meditations in yoga are better than not doing anything. However, working on your cardiovascular endurance, increasing your strength, and performing specific stretches for the muscles you use while playing soccer will provide more benefit for you than will yoga.

One additional recommendation is to avoid taking medicine to reduce your pain like Advil or Motrin (NSAID). Think about it like this; if you place your hand on a burning stove, you could leave your hand there and take medicine to reduce the pain of your hand burning. However, the smarter solution is to understand the underlying causes of your pain (the fact that your hand is on a stove) and address that (by taking your hand off the stove). **Therefore, if you ever use pain relief medicine, only use it on a very short-term basis and not as a tool for long-term pain management.**

To summarize, some things to consider besides cardio, weight training, and stretching that can improve your performance and body are:

1. Foam rolling
2. Massages
3. Percussion massage gun
4. Chiropractic care
5. Yoga

Chapter 20

Recovering from an Injury

Hopefully, you have never experienced an injury before. Hopefully, you can have a long and successful career with no injuries. However, it is much more likely that years of playing soccer will increase the chances you sustain an injury. Use the tips and guidelines in this book to help prevent injuries from occurring, but given that they may occur, let us discuss the steps to help reduce the time away from the field.

Immediately after becoming injured, the worst thing that you can do is to "play through the pain." Unless you are in the championship game of the most important game of your career, your health should be a higher priority than any single game. The more you push through the pain, the longer your recovery time will be. Therefore, playing a few more minutes of a game while injured could mean that you need to miss more games down the road.

Remember that pain is one of your body's indicators that something is wrong. Pain in your muscles is a great thing in most cases, because it means that you are breaking down your muscle fibers to rebuild them bigger and stronger later. **However, not all pain is created equal. Use pain in your soft**

tissues (i.e., spine, joints, ligaments, and tendons) as a gauge for how hard to push yourself. Some movements and exercises can seriously harm your body, so find painless alternatives to these.

Take me as an example of what not to do. I used to believe the saying, *"Pain is just weakness leaving your body."* In fact, it is still hanging in the makeshift gym in the basement of my parents' house from when I used to live there. I thought all pain was good for my body and would help me become stronger. **The problem is that breaking down muscle fibers is good pain but damaging your joints, tendons, ligaments, and spine is not good, because these parts of your body are not like muscles; they wear out and do not rebuild themselves bigger and stronger later, like muscles do.** Therefore, during every workout, make sure that you are using a full range of motion and controlled reps to avoid the injuries that so many people who weightlift experience. If you are interested in the mistakes that I made and the lessons I learned the hard way, the following is a list of injuries I had by the age of 26:

- Spine misalignment
- Upper, mid, and lower back pain
- Torn pec (chest)
- Carpal tunnel

- Multiple sprained ankles (I could not walk for three months from one)
- Strained hip flexor on my shooting leg (I could not shoot without being in pain, so I became much better with my opposite foot)
- Poor nerve function in my spine
- Biceps tendonitis

There is a Russian proverb that says a dumb person never learns from their mistakes, a smart person learns from their own mistakes, but a wise person learns from other peoples' mistakes. I have become a lot smarter, but I challenge you to be the wise person. **Care just as much about long-term health as you do momentary successes because your future self will thank you.**

Next, when you are injured, the University of Michigan Medicine Health Library suggests you use R.I.C.E—Rest, Ice, Compression, and Elevation in your recovery period immediately after the injury and for the next few weeks to reduce pain and swelling.

- **Rest** – Avoid using the injured body part which will only create more inflammation and increase the recovery time.

- **Ice** – Cold packs and ice will reduce swelling and numb the area to lessen pain so apply ice right away for 10-20 minutes each time and for as many times as you can throughout the day.

- **Compression** – Compression by wrapping the injured area with a bandage like an "Ace wrap" will help limit swelling.

- **Elevation** – Elevate the injured or sore area on pillows while applying ice and anytime you are sitting or lying down. Attempt to keep the area at or above the level of your heart to help minimize swelling.

Let us use me, a soccer player who has injured their ankle, as an example:

Rest – After injuring my ankle, I hopped on one leg to my car to avoid placing any bodyweight on the ankle.

Ice – I iced the area that night and about eight times a day for the next two months. I bought gel ice packs that did not become as cold as ice but were still cold, so I could apply them directly to my injured ankle. (Directly placing ice on an injury is often too cold.)

Compression – After I injured my ankle, I did not take my soccer cleat off until I saw a licensed physician the next day. The doctor recommended a physical therapist to aid in recovery, and he recommended a compression boot to limit the swelling.

Elevation – For the next several months, I spent a decent amount of time in a chair, in my bed, or on the couch. In all situations, I did my best to elevate my ankle above my heart to help with recovery.

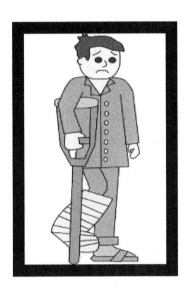

To keep muscle mass, I also used e-stim therapy on the leg that had the injured ankle. I continued working out my abdominals and upper body in the gym to ensure I retained some level of fitness during my two to three-month recovery. Additionally, because I could not play soccer for the next few months, I had the time to still workout. As mentioned previously, I obtained the advice of a licensed physician who could diagnose the torn ligaments in my ankle. **It is recommended you see a medical professional if an injury happens to you, too.**

Finally, after you have addressed your injury from the outside using R.I.C.E., help your body by providing the nutrition and anti-inflammatories to minimize your pain and speed up your recovery from the inside. In the *Understand Soccer* series book, *Soccer Nutrition*, a perfect soccer meal plan is discussed as well as when to eat each type of food to provide you more energy for games and boost recovery after the game is done. Therefore, to help with recovering more quickly so you can back on the field fast, a diet focused on fruits, vegetables, and plenty of water is the way to go. Some meat, dairy, and grains will help round out your nutrition to provide you the macronutrients and micronutrients needed to help your recovery. However, let us talk about a few key things to give your body an edge in reducing pain and reducing time away from the field.

First, fish oil has omega-3 fatty acids, which help keep your blood-fat levels in a good range. This is helpful if you are injured and need to exercise less. It also reduces stiffness, increases focus, and decreases joint pain.

Second, a study published in the *Journal of Nutritional Biochemistry* found that the oleocanthal in olive oil had a significant impact not only on chronic inflammation but also on acute inflammatory processes, like nonsteroidal anti-inflammatory drugs (NSAIDs), such as aspirin or ibuprofen (e.g., Motrin/Advil). **Therefore, you can obtain the same** inflammation-reducing properties from olive oil as you can from unnatural over-the-counter medications, which are much more likely to have negative side effects.

Third, consume some anti-inflammatory foods, like turmeric and ginger. Simply buy turmeric root and ginger root either whole or in capsule form and consume them with a meal. These two superfoods will reduce inflammation in your body, which will significantly reduce the time you need to recover. Think about the expensive medical bills that may result from your injury. Compared to that, buying and eating some ginger root and turmeric root is an inexpensive way to lessen your body's inflammation. Personally, I buy them, cut little pieces off the roots each morning, and take them like I would take a pill by washing them down with water.

In conclusion, make sure you take the time necessary to recover, do not push yourself too hard in the moment when injured, and take the necessary steps to recover.

- Aim to breakdown only the muscles when working out.
- Avoid exercises that cause spine, tendon, ligament, and joint pain.
- Avoid working out/exercising more than once per day.
- When you feel non-muscle pain, avoid continuing that exercise and consider ending all exercise that day.

- Use rest, ice, compression, and elevation.
- See a licensed medical professional to determine the extent of your injury.
- Consume foods like fish oil, olive oil, ginger, and turmeric to recover more quickly using nutrition.

Afterword

Congrats! Because you have read this book, you gained a ton of knowledge on how to improve your fitness to improve your physical abilities on the soccer field. Even more important than obtaining the knowledge from this book is that you have increased your confidence. This is huge! Just by reading this book and doing what it mentions, you give yourself a massive advantage over your competition. Knowing that you already have these advantages going into the gym and onto the field will boost your confidence. By reading this book, you have shown you care a lot about growing, and I applaud you for it. So many other players do not take a few hours to obtain the tools and information that can make fitness and all other areas of their soccer game much easier and twice as fun, but you just did. Great job! Excitingly, that is what a book can do. A book takes a person's decades of experiences, highs, lows, and knowledge and then condenses that information down into something that you can read in a few hours. Think about it, you just spent a few hours learning what took me over a decade to learn. Because of that, I know you will use the information in this book to perform like a star soccer player.

If the tips you read in this book helped you gain confidence about fitness, please leave a positive review letting me know on Amazon.com.

WAIT!

Wouldn't it be nice to have an easy one-page FREE PDF printout with off-season and in-season workouts discussed in this book? Well, here is your chance!

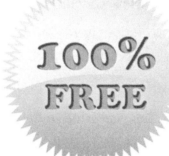

UNDERSTANDSOCCER.COM - WEIGHT TRAINING WORKOUTS

Weight Training - Off-Season

Monday - Upper Body Pull

Exercise	Sets	Reps	Workout 1	Workout 2	Workout 3
Pull-Ups	3	Max			
Rows	3	5-6			
Hip Huggers	3	5-6			
*Dumbbell Curls	3	6-8			
Leg Raises	3	Max			

Wednesday - Lower Body

Exercise	Sets	Reps	Workout 1	Workout 2	Workout 3
Bench Presses	3	5-6			
Dips	3	Max			
Overhead Presses	3	5-6			
*Triceps Extensions	3	6-8			
Sit-Ups	3	Max			

Friday - Upper Body Push

Exercise	Sets	Reps	Workout 1	Workout 2	Workout 3
Squats	3	5-8			
Deadlifts	3	5-6			
Lunges	3	6-8			
Calf Raises	3	12-15			
Planks	3	Max			

*Optional exercise for a smaller body part. Take sets to failure.
Perform a warm-up that includes warm-up sets of exercises above with reduced weight.

Weight Training - During Season

1-2X per Week

Exercise	Sets	Reps	Workout 1	Workout 2	Workout 3
Squat	2	5-6			
Deadlift	2	5-6			
Calf Raises	2	12-15			
Bench Press	2	5-6			
Pull-Ups	2	Max			
Overhead Press	2	5-6			
Rows	2	5-6			
Sit-Ups	2	Max			
Leg Raises	2	Max			

Go to this Link for an **Instant** One-Page Printout:
UnderstandSoccer.com/free-printout

This FREE workout log is simply a thank you for purchasing this book. This PDF printout will ensure that you have a terrific workout to perform to get you ready for the soccer field!

About the Author

There he was—a soccer player who had difficulties scoring. He wanted to be the best on the field but lacked the confidence and knowledge to make his goal a reality. Every day, he dreamed about improving, but the average coaching he received, combined with his lack of knowledge, only left him feeling alone and unable to attain his goal. He was a quiet player, and his performance often went unnoticed.

This all changed after his junior year on the varsity soccer team of one of the largest high schools in the state. During the team and parent banquet at the end of the season, his coach decided to say something nice about each player. When it was his turn to receive praise, the only thing that could be said was that he had scored two goals that season—even though they were against a lousy team, so they did not really count. It was a very painful statement that after the 20+ game season, all that could be said of his efforts were two goals that did not count. One of his greatest fears came true; he was called out in front of his family and friends.

Since that moment, he was forever changed. He got serious. With a new soccer mentor, he focused on training to obtain the necessary skills, build his confidence, and become the goal-scorer that he had always dreamed of being. The next season, after just a few months, he found himself moved up to the starting position of center midfielder and scored his first goal of the 26-game season in only the third game.

He continued with additional training led by a proven goal-scorer to build his knowledge. Fast-forward to the present day, and, because of the work he put in, and his focus on the necessary skills, he figured out how to become a goal-scorer who averages about two goals and an assist per game—all because he increased his understanding of how to play soccer. With the help of a soccer mentor, he took his game from being a bench-warmer who got called out in front of everybody to becoming the most confident player on the field.

Currently, he is a soccer trainer in Michigan, working for Next Level Training. He advanced through their rigorous program as a soccer player and was hired as a trainer. This program has allowed him to guide world-class soccer players for over a decade. He trains soccer players in formats ranging from one-hour classes to weeklong camps, and he instructs classes of all sizes, from groups of 30 soccer players all the way down to working one-on-one with individuals who want to play for the United States National Team.

If you enjoyed this book, then please leave a review.

Additional Books by the Author Available on Amazon:

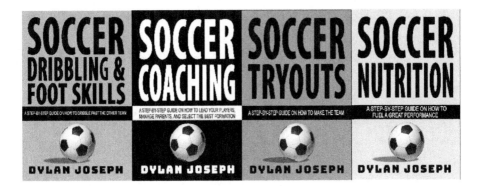

Soccer Dribbling & Foot Skills: A Step-by-Step Guide on How to Dribble Past the Other Team

Soccer Coaching: A Step-by-Step Guide on How to Lead Your Players, Manage Parents, and Select the Best Formation

Soccer Tryouts: A Step-by-Step Guide on How to Make the Team

Soccer Nutrition: A Step-by-Step Guide on How to Fuel a Great Performance

Free Book!

How would you like to get a book of your choosing in the *Understand Soccer* series for free?

Join the Soccer Squad Book Team today and receive your next book (and potentially future books) for FREE.

Signing up is easy and does not cost anything.

Check out this website for more information:

UnderstandSoccer.com/soccer-squad-book-team

Thank You for Reading!

Dear Reader,

I hope you enjoyed and learned from **Soccer Fitness**. I truly enjoyed writing these steps and tips to ensure you become strong and fast on the soccer field.

As an author, I love feedback. Candidly, you are the reason that I wrote this book and plan to write more. Therefore, tell me what you liked, what you loved, and what can be improved. I'd love to hear from you. Visit UnderstandSoccer.com and scroll to the bottom of the homepage to leave me a message in the contact section or email me at:

Dylan@UnderstandSoccer.com

Finally, I need to ask a favor. **I'd love and truly appreciate a review.**

As you likely know, reviews are a key part of my process to see whether you, the reader, enjoyed my book. The reviews allow me to write more books. You have the power to help make or break my book. Please take the 2 minutes to leave a review on Amazon.com at:

https://www.amazon.com/gp/product-review/1949511332.

In gratitude,

Dylan Joseph

Glossary

Agility - The ability to change one's body position efficiently using balance, coordination, speed, reflexes, and strength.

Ballistic Stretching - Stretches using bouncing (e.g., bouncing at the bottom of a bent over hamstring stretch to get deeper in the stretch).

Beep Test - A multi-stage fitness test used to measure cardiovascular fitness and maximum oxygen uptake (i.e., VO2 max).

Bench Press - When you lie with your back on a bench, and you press the bar and any added weight away from your body.

Body Fat Percentage - Your body fat divided by your total body mass.

Body Feint (i.e., "Feint," "Jab Step," "Fake," "Fake and Take," or "Shoulder Drop") - When you pretend to push the ball in one direction, but purposely miss, then plant with the same foot and push the ball in the other direction with the opposite foot.

Body Mass Index - A weight-to-height ratio, calculated by dividing one's weight by the square of one's height and used as an indicator of obesity for non-athletes.

Calf Raise - When you push your entire body farther up in the air by moving your ankle and pressing the floor down with the balls of your feet.

Calorie - A measure of how much energy food provides. It is the energy needed to raise the temperature of 1 gram of water through 1 °C.

Carbohydrates (i.e., "Carbs") - A macronutrient broken down by the body to provide energy from sugars, starches, and cellulose.

Cardiovascular Endurance - The ability of the heart, lungs, and blood vessels to deliver oxygen to your body tissues, so you can continue training at your current intensity.

Chiropractor - A practitioner of integrative medicine based on the diagnosis and manipulation of a misaligned spine and joints.

Circuit Training - A workout involving a series of exercises performed in rotation with minimal rest.

Conditioning - A physical fitness program to improve performance and prevent injuries.

Deadlift - In this move, a bar filled with weight is on the ground. Bend down emphasizing your leg muscles and pick up the weight while driving your hips forward.

Deload Week - A week where you limit your training to enable your body to recover fully and come back stronger afterwards.

Dynamic Stretching - Movement based stretches and warm-ups to improve performance and reduce the chance of injury (e.g., leg swings, jumping jacks, trunk rotations, and arm rotations to "loosen" up the joints and muscles).

E-Stim Therapy - Sending mild electrical pulses through the skin to help stimulate injured muscles or manipulate nerves to reduce pain.

Fats (i.e., "Lipids") - A macronutrient to provide your body energy, support cell growth, protect your organs, keep your body warm, absorb fat-soluble nutrients, and produce important hormones.

Fat-Soluble Vitamins - Vitamins A, D, E, and K that dissolve in fat and oils. They can be stored in the body's fat stores.

Fitness - Being physically fit and healthy.

Flexibility - Bending easily without breaking.

Foam Rolling - A muscle release technique used to eliminate muscle restrictions by rolling on a cylinder.

High-Intensity Interval Training (i.e., "HIIT") - Alternating short periods of intense exercise with recovery periods.

Inflammation - The immune system's response to injury and infection to tell the immune system to heal and repair damaged tissue, as well as defend itself against foreign invaders, such as viruses and bacteria.

Joint - The area where two bones are connected to enable body parts to move. These are usually formed of fibrous connective tissue and cartilage.

Ketosis - When your body uses fat as your primary fuel for energy after all the carbohydrates have been used in your system.

Keystone Habit - Routines that automatically lead to multiple positive behaviors and positive effects in your life.

Leg Press - While sitting in a leg press machine, use your leg muscles to push the platform.

Ligament - A short band of tough, flexible fibrous connective tissue which connects two bones or cartilages or holds together a joint.

Lunge - Extending one leg in front of your body and one leg behind your body, and then lowering your body into a half-squat with just the one leg forward.

Macronutrition - Fats, proteins, and carbohydrates needed in large amounts in your diet.

Mindset - The established set of attitudes and beliefs held by someone.

Moving First Touch (i.e., "Attacking Touch") - Pushing the ball into space with your first touch, which is the opposite of taking a touch where the ball stops underneath you (i.e., at your feet).

Multi-Joint/Compound Exercise - An exercise that works multiple muscle groups at the same time (e.g., a squat or deadlift).

Muscular Endurance - The ability of a muscle or group of muscles to sustain repeated contractions against resistance for an extended period.

Muscular Strength - The amount of force a muscle can produce with a single maximal effort.

Nutrition - Food necessary for health and growth.

Omega-3 Fatty Acids - An unsaturated fatty acid occurring in fish oil that helps with brain development, joint health, and good skin.

Plank - Extending your arms straight out (i.e., at the top of the push-up position) or planting your forearms and elbows on the ground while keeping your body straight.

Plyometrics - Exercise involving repeated rapid stretching and contracting of muscles by jumping to increase muscle power.

Power - The ability to move weight with speed.

Protein - A macronutrient made up of many amino acids that help aid in normal cell function, muscle growth, creating enzymes, producing hormones, and can be used for energy, too.

Pull-Up - When you are hanging from a bar and pull your chin up and over the bar.

Push-Up - When your hands and body are prone on the floor, and you push your body up using your chest, shoulders, and triceps.

R.I.C.E. - Rest, ice, compression, and elevation to reduce injuries.

Routine - A sequence of actions regularly followed.

Self-Pass (i.e., "L," "Iniesta," or "La Croqueta") - Passing the ball from one foot to the other while running. Imagine you are doing a roll, but without your foot going on top of the ball. Instead, it is an inside of the foot pass from one foot and an inside of the foot push up the field with the other foot.

Single-Joint/Isolation Exercise - An exercise engaging a single muscle group within the body (e.g., leg curl, biceps curl, and quadriceps extension).

Sit-Up - When you use your abdominals to raise your upper body up.

Speed - The rate at which someone can move.

Squat - For this move, the bar is on your back while you are squatting down and then standing up again using your hips, quadriceps, hamstrings, and glutes.

Static Stretching - Holding a stretch for 20-60 seconds to promote recovery and increase your flexibility (e.g., holding a bent over hamstring stretch where you try to touch your toes without bouncing, but with each exhale, you go deeper into the stretch).

Stretching - The activity done before physical activity to help prepare you and performed after physical activity to help recovery.

Superman - Exercise where you lie prone on your stomach. Extend your legs behind you and raise your arms into the air.

Tendon - A flexible but inelastic cord of strong fibrous collagen tissue attaching a muscle to a bone.

Warm-Up - The time spent prior to your practice or game where you are "warming" your body up by using dynamic stretches and moves to mimic what you will be doing while playing.

Vitamins – Necessary for energy production, immune function, blood clotting, and other functions.

Water-Soluble Vitamins - Vitamins B and C are not stored in the body, so they must be taken in daily.

Weight Training - Physical training that involves lifting weights.

Acknowledgments

I would like to thank you, the reader. I am grateful to provide you value and to help you on your journey of becoming a fitter soccer player. I am happy to serve you and thank you for the opportunity to do so. Also, I would like to recognize people that have made a difference and have paved the way for me to share this book with you:

I want to thank the grammar editor, Abbey Decker. Her terrific understanding of the complexities of the English language ensured that the wording needed to convey the messages was appropriate and she provided countless grammatical improvements.

Also, I would like to thank the content editors Kevin Solorio, Toni Sinistaj, and Youssef Hodroj. They reviewed this book for areas that could be improved and additional insights to share that could immediately help you, the reader.

Many thanks,

Dylan Joseph

Printed in Great Britain
by Amazon

31745138R00069